CONTINGENCY MANAGEMENT FOR ADOLESCENT SUBSTANCE ABUSE

Contingency Management for Adolescent Substance Abuse

A PRACTITIONER'S GUIDE

Scott W. Henggeler
Phillippe B. Cunningham
Melisa D. Rowland
Sonja K. Schoenwald
and Associates

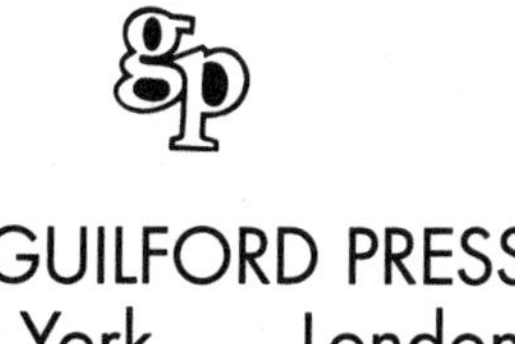

THE GUILFORD PRESS
New York London

A Division of Guilford Publications, Inc.
72 Spring Street, New York, NY 10012
www.guilford.com

Printed in the United States of America

This book is printed on acid-free paper.

Last digit is print number: 9 8 7 6 5 4 3 2 1

The authors have checked with sources believed to be reliable in their efforts to provide information that is complete and generally in accord with the standards of practice that are accepted at the time of publication. However, in view of the possibility of human error or changes in behavioral, mental health, or medical sciences, neither the authors, nor the editor and publisher, nor any other party who has been involved in the preparation or publication of this work warrants that the information contained herein is in every respect accurate or complete, and they are not responsible for any errors or omissions or the results obtained from the use of such information. Readers are encouraged to confirm the information contained in this book with other sources.

Library of Congress Cataloging-in-Publication Data

Contingency management for adolescent substance abuse : a practitioner's guide / by Scott W. Henggeler . . . [et al.].
p. cm.
Includes bibliographical references and index.
ISBN 978-1-4625-0247-9 (pbk.: alk. paper)
1. Teenagers—Substance use. 2. Substance abuse—Treatment—Handbooks, manuals, etc. 3. Cognitive therapy—Handbooks, manuals, etc. I. Henggeler, Scott W., 1950–
HV4999.Y68C67 2012
616.86′06—dc23

2011037659

About the Authors

Scott W. Henggeler, PhD, is Professor of Psychiatry and Behavioral Sciences and Director of the Family Services Research Center (FSRC) at the Medical University of South Carolina in Charleston. The mission of the FSRC is to develop, validate, and study the dissemination of clinically- and cost-effective mental health and substance abuse services for children with serious clinical problems and their families. Dr. Henggeler has published 10 books and more than 250 journal articles and book chapters, and has received grants from several foundations and government agencies. He is Associate Editor of the *Journal of Consulting and Clinical Psychology*, has been on the editorial boards of more than 10 journals, and is on the board of the National Association of Drug Court Professionals.

Phillippe B. Cunningham, PhD, is Professor of Psychiatry and Behavioral Sciences in the FSRC at the Medical University of South Carolina. He has had a longstanding commitment to addressing the psychosocial needs of children and adolescents, especially those who are disadvantaged and underserved. In 2000 Dr. Cunningham received the Theodore H. Blau Early Career Award from the American Psychological Association's Society of Clinical Psychology, and in 2006 he participated in the First Lady's Conference on Helping America's Youth.

Melisa D. Rowland, MD, is Associate Professor of Psychiatry and Behavioral Sciences in the FSRC at the Medical University of South Carolina. Dr. Rowland's research interests focus on developing, implementing, and evaluating clinically effective family-based interventions for youth who present serious emotional and behavioral problems. She is the co-investigator of clinical and project implementation on a study funded by the National Institute on Drug Abuse that evaluates the relative effectiveness of three training protocols with increasing intensity in supporting the implementation of contingency management by practitioners treating adolescent substance abusers in the South Carolina mental health and substance abuse sectors. Dr. Rowland is also the co-investigator of clinical implementation for an Annie E. Casey Foundation–funded project designed to develop an evidence-based continuum of services for New York City youth with antisocial behaviors at risk of out-of-home placement.

Sonja K. Schoenwald, PhD, is Professor of Psychiatry and Behavioral Sciences in the FSRC at the Medical University of South Carolina. She is among the leading clinical services researchers in the country on issues relating to the transportability, implementation, and dissemination of effective community-based treatments for youth with serious clinical problems and their families. Dr. Schoenwald pioneered the development, refinement, and empirical testing of the quality assurance protocols used to adapt multisystemic therapy (MST) for juvenile offenders and their families to diverse communities. She has published numerous peer-reviewed papers and book chapters and has coauthored three books and several treatment manuals and monographs on the implementation of effective treatments in communities nationally and internationally.

Cynthia Cupit Swenson, PhD, is Professor of Psychiatry and Behavioral Sciences and Associate Director of the FSRC at the Medical University of South Carolina. She is a developer of MST for a child abuse and neglect treatment model based on a 5-year randomized clinical trial funded by the National Institute of Mental Health. She is currently Principal Investigator on a study funded by the National Institute on Drug Abuse that evaluates a family-based treatment model for co-occurring parental substance abuse and child maltreatment. Dr. Swenson has conducted research in the child abuse and neglect area nationally and internationally for 20 years.

Ashli J. Sheidow, PhD, is Associate Professor of Psychiatry and Behavioral Sciences in the FSRC at the Medical University of South Carolina. Dr. Sheidow's research interests have focused broadly on the development, prevention, and treatment of adolescent psychopathology and juvenile delinquency from an ecological perspective, with concentrations in co-occurring disorders, effective dissemination of evidence-based practices, and advanced quantitative methods.

Michael R. McCart, PhD, is Assistant Professor of Psychiatry and Behavioral Sciences in the FSRC at the Medical University of South Carolina. His research interests focus on the development, evaluation, and dissemination of evidence-based interventions for substance abuse, disruptive behavior disorders, and posttraumatic stress disorder among adolescents. Dr. McCart has received awards from the U.S. Department of Justice and the American Professional Society on the Abuse of Children for his clinical work with adolescents and their families.

Brad Donohue, PhD, is Professor in the Psychology Department at the University of Nevada, Las Vegas (UNLV), and Co-Editor of the *Journal of Child and Adolescent Substance Abuse.* His primary research interests are the development, evaluation, and dissemination of evidence-based treatments, including MST and family behavior therapy.

Dr. Donohue is coauthor of the books *Treating Adult Substance Abuse Using Family Behavior Therapy* and *Treating Adolescent Substance Abuse Using Family Behavior Therapy*. He has received several awards for his research at UNLV.

Ligia A. Navas-Murphy, MS, has had over 8 years' experience working as a therapist in the mental health field. Focusing on the treatment of children, adolescents, and families with various needs, she has provided in-home and outpatient clinic-based treatment. Dr. Navas-Murphy established Palmetto Advocacy for Children, LLC, in Murrells Inlet, South Carolina, an agency that provides assistance and guidance to parents during the process of obtaining appropriate and effective services to meet their children's needs.

Jeff Randall, PhD, is Assistant Professor of Psychiatry and Behavioral Sciences in the FSRC at the Medical University of South Carolina. He was the director of a randomized clinical trial of juvenile drug courts and MST funded by the National Institute on Drug Abuse and the National Institue on Alcohol Abuse and Alcoholism. Dr Randall's research interests include MST conceptualization, implementation, and treatment; adolescent substance abuse; juvenile drug courts; and anxiety disorders.

Preface

The material in this manual has been developed and refined by a group of clinician investigators funded by the National Institute on Drug Abuse to improve the availability and delivery of evidence-based treatments to youth who abuse drugs. Earlier versions of this book (Cunningham et al., 2002, 2004; Family Services Research Center, 2008a, 2008b) were available only to our collaborators in studies designed to help community-based therapists use contingency management (CM) to treat adolescent substance abuse. The present book represents our distilled learning modified through many years of experience training and consulting with hundreds of therapists attempting to implement CM with integrity. We are very pleased that this work is now available to a broader audience.

Contents

CHAPTER 1

Introduction to Contingency Management

GOAL OF THIS BOOK

The overriding purpose of this treatment manual is to provide practitioners with straightforward, user-friendly, and detailed guidelines for implementing contingency management (CM) with substance-abusing adolescents. Although CM is one of the most extensively researched and best validated interventions in the field of substance abuse treatment, it is rarely used in treating adolescents. This book aims to narrow the gap between what has been proven to be effective (i.e., CM as an evidence-based treatment) and what is practiced in clinical settings—with the ultimate purpose of improving outcomes for substance-abusing youth.

Several features of CM support its viability for widespread adoption by clinicians who treat adolescents.

1. Most important, and as detailed subsequently, CM and its variations have proven effective in treating substance abuse in adults, and results from several controlled studies support its promise in treating substance abuse in adolescents.
2. The clinical techniques used in CM are based on cognitive-behavioral and behavior therapy principles, and therapist attitudes toward these types of intervention strategies are relatively positive (Henggeler et al., 2007). Favorable attitudes enhance the adoptability of CM by practitioners working in community settings.
3. Also enhancing the adoptability of CM is its capacity to be adapted for use in a variety of outpatient treatment environments, including family therapy and individual therapy with parental involvement. Thus, therapists are not necessarily required to change their preferred methods of delivering treatment.
4. Importantly, CM is also much easier to adopt than are other evidence-based treatments of adolescent substance abuse such as multisystemic therapy (MST),

multidimensional family therapy, and brief strategic family therapy. Although effective, these family therapy approaches require considerable hands-on training by purveyor organizations, ongoing quality assurance to support treatment fidelity, and full-time therapists dedicated solely to the particular approach, all of which can be costly and are challenging to implement. CM, on the other hand, can be delivered by practitioners from varying backgrounds and theoretical perspectives.

In sum, CM is an evidence-based substance abuse treatment that can be integrated into the regular clinical practice of therapists who work with adolescents. The remainder of this chapter provides further support for the viability of CM in outpatient settings.

RISK FACTORS FOR SUBSTANCE ABUSE AND HOW THEY ARE ADDRESSED BY CM

Reviewers have identified a relatively consistent set of malleable factors (i.e., variables that can be influenced by treatment) that are associated with adolescent substance use and abuse (e.g., Loeber, Farrington, Stouthamer-Loeber, & Van Kammen, 1998; Schaeffer, Chang, & Henggeler, 2009; Tarter, Vanyukov, & Kirisci, 2008). These factors pertain primarily to the characteristics of adolescents and the social systems in which they are embedded.

- At the *individual level*, substance use is associated with positive attitudes toward problem behavior and substance use, emotional problems, and social skill deficits.
- At the *family level*, low caregiver supervision and inconsistent discipline are important correlates.
- Most significantly, however, association with *substance-using peers* is a consistently powerful predictor of adolescent substance use.

These correlates have important implications for treatment. Indeed, the leading evidence-based treatments of serious antisocial behavior in adolescents specifically address these key risk factors comprehensively (Henggeler & Sheidow, 2011).

CM also addresses a range of important risk factors.

- On an *individual level*, for example (see Chapter 5), the therapist works with the youth and parent to help the youth develop and manage situations that have previously led to substance use. Similarly, the adolescent is helped to develop drug refusal skills for those high-risk situations that are unavoidable.
- Regarding *family risk factors*, caregivers are critical to virtually all components of CM implementation: determining the need for treatment (Chapter 2), identifying situations and persons that put the youth at risk for using substances (Chapter 4), developing plans to avoid and cope with high-risk situations (Chapter 5), urine

testing to track substance use (Chapter 7), and providing incentives for abstinence (Chapter 6). Together, this involvement in the treatment and monitoring of performance necessarily increases parental supervision and the consistency of discipline.

- Finally, the critical role of association with *substance-using peers* is addressed as well. As situations that place the youth at risk for substance use are identified and examined in detail (Chapter 4), certain of the youth's peers are almost always identified as contributing to his or her substance use. Subsequently, plans are made to decrease these peer contacts (Chapters 5 and 6), and the implementation of these plans is tracked closely.

Thus, CM incorporates a relatively comprehensive framework in attenuating the negative effects of substance use risk factors while building protective factors such as social skills, family involvement, and contacts with prosocial peers.

THE EVIDENCE BASE FOR CM

Reviews of CM in the adult drug abuse treatment literature (e.g., Higgins, Silverman, & Heil, 2008; National Institute on Drug Abuse, 2009; Petry, 2000; Roozen et al., 2004) clearly indicate that a behavior therapy approach that includes close monitoring of substance use can be regarded as effective. Higgins and Budney (Budney & Higgins, 1998; Higgins & Budney, 1993), for example, developed a behavioral treatment protocol (community reinforcement approach) for adult drug abusers that includes a voucher system linked with results from frequent urine analyses, functional analysis of drug use, and development of drug refusal skills. Their model has proven effective with adult cocaine abusers (e.g., Higgins et al., 2003) and has also been examined with adults in treatment for opiate dependence (e.g., Bickel, Amass, Higgins, Badger, & Esch, 1997) and alcohol dependence (e.g., Petry, Martin, Cooney, & Kranzler, 2000).

Regarding treatment of adolescent substance abuse, an early variation of CM developed by Azrin, Donohue, and colleagues has produced promising results in several studies (Azrin et al., 1996; Azrin, Donohue, Besalel, Kogan, & Acierno, 1994; Azrin, McMahon, et al., 1994; Donohue & Azrin, 2001). Subsequently, findings from our randomized trial with substance-abusing juvenile offenders in juvenile drug court (Henggeler et al., 2006) showed that the integration of evidence-based treatments (i.e., MST and CM) improved standard drug court outcomes for substance use. Moreover, the integration of CM accelerated the decrease in substance use achieved by MST. Finally, using an approach similar to that of the present manual, Stanger, Budney, Kamon, and Thostensen (2009) completed a randomized trial of CM with marijuana-using adolescents and showed promising results at posttreatment. In conclusion, extensive findings with adults and emerging findings for adolescents (Stanger & Budney, 2010) support the effectiveness of CM, and the reader is referred to the literature reviews and studies cited previously for more extensive information on the capacity of CM to reduce substance use.

OVERVIEW OF CM CLINICAL PROCEDURES

CM is based on and integrates therapeutic interventions from two widely used clinical models: behavioral therapy and cognitive-behavioral therapy (CBT). In addition to the use of these strategies in the treatment of substance use, as cited previously, behavioral therapies and CBTs have been widely supported in the treatment of a variety of mental health problems experienced by children and adolescents (Weisz & Kazdin, 2010). In CM, behavioral interventions are critical for reinforcing desired changes in youth behavior. For example, the therapist and caregivers arrange a system in which clean urine screens are rewarded with privileges and resources that are highly desired by the youth (see Chapter 6), whereas dirty screens are met with consequences that are unpleasant but socially useful. The cognitive-behavioral interventions used in CM largely address social skill and problem-solving skill deficits in the adolescent that increase the risk of drug use. For example, the youth, with support from the therapist and caregivers, will learn to identify situations in which drug use is likely and develop strategies for coping effectively with those situations.

The chapters are presented in a sequence that corresponds to their use in clinical practice.

1. ***Determining the Need for Substance Use Treatment (Chapter 2).*** Specific guidelines and well-validated assessment instruments are provided to assist the therapist in determining whether the youth's substance use is largely experimental in nature and, therefore, does not necessarily require interventions, or whether the youth's substance use suggests abuse or dependence, which reflects more serious problems and likely requires therapeutic interventions.

2. ***Introducing Contingency Management and Engaging Families in Treatment (Chapter 3).*** An overview of CM is provided to orient the youth and caregivers to the treatment process. In addition, as the importance of caregiver involvement has been clearly established in the adolescent substance abuse treatment literature (Waldron & Turner, 2008; Williams & Chang, 2000), guidelines are presented for engaging the family to support the youth's substance abuse treatment. These guidelines are based, in part, on the effective strategies (i.e., 98% treatment completion rate) used to engage families of substance-abusing youths in MST (Henggeler, Pickrel, Brondino, & Crouch, 1996).

3. ***ABC Assessment of Drug Use (Chapter 4).*** All treatment planning is individualized to the specific circumstances of each youth's substance use. The times, places, situations, persons, thoughts, and feelings that accompany substance use are identified; and these, along with an analysis of the consequences, provide the bases for subsequent clinical decision making by the therapist, youth, and caregivers. Together, the integration of these contributing circumstances, drug use behaviors, and outcomes for the youth constitute the ABC assessment: antecedents, behaviors, and consequences.

4. ***Self-Management Planning and Drug Refusal Skills Training (Chapter 5).*** Based on the results of the ABC assessment, cognitive-behavioral strategies are individualized to the specific circumstances of the youth's substance use. The therapist and caregivers

help the youth develop strategies to avoid high-risk situations and to cope with risky situations that are unavoidable. The success of these strategies is reviewed during each treatment session, self-management plans are revised as needed, and subsequent outcomes are reassessed until effectiveness is achieved.

5. ***The Point-and-Level Reward System (Chapter 6).*** The therapist guides the youth and caregivers in developing a point-and-level system that details incentives (e.g., rewards and privileges) for clean drug and alcohol tests and disincentives (e.g., extra chores) for dirty drug and alcohol screens. This behavior therapy approach aims to reinforce desired youth behavior and appropriately punish undesired behavior. Contingencies are modified as treatment progresses.

6. ***Drug Testing Protocol (Chapter 7).*** Drug testing through random urine drug screens and alcohol breath tests is used to objectively monitor the effectiveness of the CM interventions. Results from such testing also serve as the basis for providing the youth with rewards for not using drugs. The therapist teaches the caregivers to conduct the urine screens at home using procedures that yield valid results.

7. ***Synthesizing the Components of Contingency Management (Chapter 8).*** Once youth and caregivers have practiced the various aspects of CM, therapists begin to combine all components into each treatment session. This chapter provides a guide for integrating the behavioral (drug screens, contract, reward menu) and cognitive-behavioral (ABC assessment, self-management planning, drug refusal skills) aspects of CM as treatment progresses. Strategies to help youth and families sustain clinical gains following CM are reviewed.

8. ***Conducting Contingency Management without Caregivers (Chapter 9).*** Because caregivers may be temporarily or permanently absent from CM sessions, strategies for conducting CM without them are reviewed. A modified contract and template for developing a reward menu are also provided.

Who Is Appropriate for CM Interventions and What about the Parents?

This treatment manual is intended for use with 12- to 17-year-old adolescents who (1) are abusing substances as delineated in Chapter 2 and (2) are living with their biological (e.g., parents, grandparents, other adult family members), adoptive, or foster family caregivers. The CM substance abuse interventions are appropriate for youth with co-occurring problems (e.g., delinquency, depression), assuming that these problems are also being addressed during treatment. The most important characteristics of the participating caregiver are that he or she has a genuine concern for the welfare of the youth and possesses sufficient influence in the family to collaborate with, specify (e.g., contingency contract), and enforce (e.g., collect drug screens, apply contingencies) the components of the CM treatment protocol. Thus, the interventions described within this manual are applicable to a broad range of substance-abusing adolescents, but they are not intended for delivery in residential treatment contexts (e.g., residential treatment centers, inpatient programs, boot camps, group homes).

Therapist Qualifications

This treatment manual is intended for use by clinical professionals with formal training in counseling, social work, family therapy, psychology or psychiatry that work in outpatient, home-, or community-based settings in the public, academic, or private sectors. Indeed, research transporting CM to community-based practitioners has demonstrated widespread interest in CM (Henggeler et al., 2007; Henggeler, Chapman, et al., 2008). Ideally, professionals interested in using CM should have prior knowledge of cognitive-behavioral and behavioral interventions as well as experience working with youth and families. The manual is not intended for use by professionals without formal clinical training (e.g., probation officers, teachers) or by those working in residential or group treatment contexts.

The Structure of Treatment over Time

The CM intervention protocol is generally applied in a straightforward manner that follows the sequence of chapters, but timing and duration of treatment and the frequency of sessions can be flexed to youth and family needs. For example, in a case in which substance abuse is the most critical presenting problem and sessions are conducted weekly, the first session might be devoted to determining the need for treatment (Chapter 2), the second to introducing CM and engaging the youth and caregivers (Chapter 3), and the third and fourth to the ABC assessment and teaching the youth and caregivers how to develop and implement self-management plans and practice drug refusal skills (Chapters 4 and 5). Subsequent sessions would focus on developing an individualized reward menu based on the point-and-level system, signing a contract, and training the parents to collect urine drug screens and alcohol breath tests (Chapters 6 and 7). Optimally, once families have practiced each component of CM and the framework of a contract and reward menu is in place, subsequent sessions involve an integrated approach in which each aspect of CM is reviewed and implemented as needed (Chapter 8). These sessions are often used to monitor and adjust ongoing behavioral (e.g., reward menu) or cognitive-behavioral (e.g., self-management plans) aspects of treatment based on outcomes (e.g., dirty screen, difficulty implementing drug refusal skills). On average, the typical course of treatment might last 14 to 18 weeks.

On the other hand, circumstances might emerge in which treatment can be expedited (e.g., substance abuse treatment is the clear focus, more than one session per week is possible, youth responds quickly to interventions), and the entire CM protocol might be completed in fewer than 14 weeks. Alternatively, the length of treatment will likely be longer in situations where significant co-occurring problems are being treated simultaneously, challenges are being faced in family engagement, clinical progress is slow, or sessions are being missed or scheduled infrequently. Here the sequence and process of protocol implementation should remain the same, but efficiency and results might be diminished. Regardless of the rate at which youth and families are progressing in CM, it is always critical to track outcomes consistently and adjust interventions based on these results.

Which Drugs Does CM Target?

Cannabis is by far the most widely abused substance by adolescents in the United States (Johnston, O'Malley, Bachman, & Schulenberg, 2007), and the examples in this manual focus primarily on marijuana abuse. CM interventions, however, are effective for a broad range of substances, including alcohol and cocaine. In general, CM can be used to treat a drug of abuse as long as that drug can be reliably and routinely detected by urine screens, breath scans, or other scientifically proven methods. As such, the language describing CM throughout this book uses the more generic terms of substance abuse and drug abuse.

OVERCOMING POTENTIAL ADMINISTRATIVE BARRIERS TO IMPLEMENTING CM

The CM approach presented in this manual is designed to overcome the most commonly encountered barriers to implementing CM. Barriers that pertain to clinical challenges are described throughout subsequent chapters, with corresponding suggestions for overcoming them. Here barriers that pertain to the organization in which the therapist works are discussed.

No Funds Are Available to Provide Vouchers or Incentives for Clean Urine Drug Screens

Such funds are desired, but are not necessary to implement CM. Chapter 6 describes how therapists can help families find indigenous family- and community-based resources to reward abstinence. This chapter also provides information on how to implement the point-and-level system used in CM without the use of vouchers or gift rewards that are external to the family's ecology.

The Collection of Drug Urine Drug Screens Is Prohibited in the Clinic

Chapter 7 details procedures to teach parents how to collect and interpret the results of urine drug screens. Thus, the point-and-level system component of CM, as described in Chapter 6, can still be fully implemented.

Expert Supervision Is Not Available When Therapists Get "Stuck" on Various Components of CM

Many practitioners do not have supervisory support for clinical implementation challenges, and for those who have such support, the supervisor might or might not be proficient in family, behavioral, and cognitive-behavioral interventions. Through extensive experience in training practitioners and supervising the implementation of CM, we have identified the most commonly experienced challenges and provided troubleshooting tips in each chapter.

The Practitioner Provides Only Individual or Family Therapy

One of the major advantages of CM is its capacity to be used in a variety of outpatient treatment environments, including family therapy and individual therapy. For example, CM has been successfully integrated into MST (e.g., Henggeler, Sheidow, Cunningham, Donohue, & Ford, 2008), juvenile drug court (e.g., Henggeler, McCart, Cunningham, & Chapman, 2011), and individual therapy contexts (Henggeler, Chapman, et al., 2008). Thus, therapists are not necessarily required to change their preferred or required methods of delivering treatment.

CM Is Too Complicated to Implement

We have aimed to provide a straightforward and detailed description of the many logical steps in the implementation of CM. To facilitate this process, chapters include conceptual overviews, checklists for each step in the intervention, forms to support the process, troubleshooting tips, handouts, and sample dialogues. Together, we hope that these resources are sufficient to support effective implementation in the vast majority of cases.

What about Implementing CM in Group Therapy?

Although Waldron and Turner (2008) concluded that group-based CBT has solid evidence for effectiveness, other researchers have concluded that any intervention that places high-risk youth in prolonged contact with each other risks detrimental effects. This latter conclusion is based on the extensive documentation of peer contagion by Dodge, Dishion, and Lansford (2006), numerous well-designed longitudinal studies showing association with deviant peers to be a powerful predictor of serious antisocial behavior in high-risk youth (Liberman, 2008), and meditational studies showing the important roles of improved family relations and decreased association with deviant peers in reducing the antisocial behavior of juvenile offenders (Eddy & Chamberlain, 2000; Huey, Henggeler, Brondino, & Pickrel, 2000), including those in juvenile drug courts (Schaeffer et al., 2010). Thus, we do not recommend implementing CM within a group therapy context, and the manual is not written to support such.

Agency Staff Are Concerned about "Rewarding" Youth to Stay Clean

In Chapter 6 we suggest strategies for addressing concerns from caregivers about rewarding youth for abstaining from substance use. With regard to agency staff, few of the more than 400 mental health and substance abuse therapists surveyed in our CM adoption and implementation study (Henggeler et al., 2007; Henggeler, Chapman, et al., 2008) reported negative views regarding use of incentives to promote youth abstinence.

ORGANIZATION OF THE CHAPTERS

Chapters 2 through 8 are organized in the following manner:

1. ***Therapist Goals***—provides an outline of therapeutic tasks that are subsequently described in detail.
2. ***Overview***—explains how the specific therapist goals for the chapter fit into the broader context of CM and gives practical information specific to the goals.
3. ***Specific Therapist Tasks***—presents in depth each of the tasks listed in the Therapist Goals section (1).
   a. ***Objectives*** corresponding to the task are described.
   b. ***Materials*** needed to accomplish the task are listed. These include session checklists for each task that can be used as a template for therapy as well as forms and handouts to facilitate the treatment process.
   c. ***Accomplishing the Objectives*** provides a discussion of how to carry out objectives.
   d. ***Troubleshooting Tips*** presents suggestions for dealing with commonly encountered problems.
   e. ***Therapist Checklists, Forms, and Handouts*** listed in the Materials section are provided near the end of the chapter.
   f. ***A Sample Dialogue*** of a therapist completing the tasks outlined in the chapter is provided.

Chapter 9 provides suggestions for managing the therapist's primary CM implementation tasks when caregivers are occasionally or permanently absent from the treatment sessions. The structure of this chapter is similar to that of Chapters 2 through 8: Therapist goals, overviews, tasks, and some substitute forms and handouts are provided.

The remainder of the book is structured to provide the conceptual information, clinical details, and materials needed to implement CM effectively. However, it is first essential to determine whether a clinical intervention for substance abuse is warranted. Chapter 2 describes how to assess a youth's substance use, its possible impact on his or her psychosocial functioning, and the corresponding need for treatment.

CHAPTER 2

Determining the Need for Substance Use Treatment

THERAPIST GOALS

1. **Determine the extent to which the youth is using substances.**
2. **Determine the impact of the youth's drug use and need for treatment.**

The purpose of this chapter is to provide therapists with information concerning how to assess youth for substance use and determine whether a clinical intervention is warranted.

OVERVIEW OF DETERMINING WHETHER THE YOUTH NEEDS SUBSTANCE USE TREATMENT

This chapter describes how therapists can assess whether a youth currently has a substance use problem that warrants clinical interventions (i.e., CM). First, however, a frame of reference is provided for understanding the important distinctions among substance use, abuse, and dependence and the role of the "referral problems" in facilitating these determinations.

A Continuum of Drug Use: From Abstinence to Dependence

Winters, Latimer, and Stinchfield (2001) provide an excellent framework for conceptualizing the continuum from substance abstinence to dependence and for understanding the factors that must be considered in placing a particular youth along this continuum. Drawing from a report by the Center for Substance Abuse Treatment (1999), the 5-point continuum includes:

1. *Abstinence*—no substance use.
2. *Experimental use*—typically minimal use in the context of recreational activities.
3. *Early abuse*—more established use, greater frequency of use, often more than one drug used, negative consequences of use beginning to emerge.
4. *Abuse*—history of frequent use, negative consequences have emerged.
5. *Dependence*—continued regular use in spite of negative consequences, considerable activity devoted to seeking and using drugs.

As noted in epidemiological studies, the majority of adolescents have used substances. Hence, substance use by itself is rarely a criterion for intervention. Rather, treatment should be reserved for youth at the early abuse, abuse, and dependence points on the continuum. Importantly, Winters and colleagues noted that several additional factors should be considered in deciding whether interventions are warranted.

1. Use of some drugs (e.g., heroin) is sufficiently dangerous as to merit intervention even if negative consequences have not emerged.
2. Age should be considered. For example, a 12-year-old experimenting with marijuana may present a very different profile than a 17-year-old with similar use.
3. Acute ingestion of large quantities of a substance at any age is sufficiently risky as to call for interventions.
4. Use of substances in inappropriate settings (e.g., at school, while driving) might justify interventions.

Thus, the general rule for deciding whether interventions for substance use are needed is based on an observed link between substance use and negative life outcomes or high risk for such outcomes. For example, youth whose substance use puts them at risk for arrest, probation, poor school performance, or family difficulties would be candidates for intervention.

Substance Use Is an Identified Referral Problem

The most obvious indicator that a youth might have a drug problem is that he or she was referred specifically for substance abuse treatment. Once in a great while, a youth might voluntarily seek treatment for substance use. More often, however, youth are referred for treatment because a caregiver suspects or has confirmed that the youth uses drugs, or because another agency involved in the life of the youth and family, such as the juvenile court, suspects or has confirmed such use. Even when the youth is referred specifically for substance use treatment, however, it is important to assess whether drug use is currently ongoing and problematic. The impact of the drug use on the youth's functioning should be assessed in key domains of life—at home, in school, with peers, and in the broader community. A worksheet is provided (*Domains of Functioning* [Form 2.4]) later in this chapter to assist with this process.

Substance Use Is Not an Identified Referral Problem

Youth receiving mental health or juvenile justice services are at increased risk for co-occurring substance abuse or dependence. Thus, many youth with behavioral or emotional problems also have undetected drug use problems. When treating youth referred for problems other than drug use, several kinds of experiences might prompt therapists to assess whether the youth is also using drugs, among them:

1. You hear, see, or smell something that makes you wonder whether the youth uses or has friends who use drugs (e.g., you smell marijuana on a youth's jacket, youth seems "spacey" and tired).
2. Someone else thinks the youth or his or her friends use drugs (e.g., in a family session, the parent expresses disapproval of a new boyfriend, saying she thinks he uses drugs).
3. Treatment goals are not being met, and you suspect drug use is one factor contributing to the lack of progress.

Aims and Time Frame of the Following Task

The primary goals for this chapter are to determine the extent to which a youth is using substances and the impact of that substance use on the youth's functioning. Based on this information, the therapist then helps the youth and caregiver determine the need for further treatment. The amount of time needed to accomplish these goals will vary greatly depending on the severity of substance use and the family's conceptualization of its impact on youth and family functioning. Families for whom drug use is not a primary presenting problem may need a full-hour session or more with the therapist to determine whether a substance abuse intervention is needed, while others might already be aware of the severity of the problem and complete the assessment form (*Substance Use Chart* [Form 2.3]) within a few minutes.

THERAPIST TASK 2.1: ASSESSING YOUTH SUBSTANCE USE AND THE NEED FOR TREATMENT

Objectives

1. Determine the extent to which the youth is using substances.
2. Determine the impact of the youth's drug use and need for treatment.

Materials

- *Therapist Flowchart and Checklist 2.1: Determining the Need for Substance Use Treatment*
- *Modified CAGE Questionnaire* (Form 2.1)
- *Client Substance Index—Short Form* (Form 2.2)

- *Substance Use Chart* (Form 2.3)
- *Domains of Functioning* (Form 2.4)
- *Common Symptoms of Drug Use* (Handout 2.1)
- *Commonly Abused Drugs Chart* (Handout 2.2)

Accomplishing the Objectives

The primary goal is to determine whether the youth's substance use is linked with problems functioning in family, peer, school, or community contexts and thus indicates a need for substance abuse treatment.

Assess Substance Use.

As presented in *Therapist Flowchart and Checklist 2.1: Determining the Need for Substance Use Treatment*, the first step is to clarify whether the presenting problems include substance use. If substance use is a presenting problem, the therapist proceeds to gather information on the youth's substance use. If drug use is not a presenting problem but is suspected as a contributing factor to other presenting problems (e.g., arrests, school difficulties), suggestions are made for determining whether more extensive substance use evaluation is needed.

When trying to determine whether a youth has substance abuse problems, it is important to obtain current and past information from multiple informants in the youth's ecology. This might include observing and interviewing the youth as well as getting information from the caregivers and other potential sources such as teachers or school records, past clinical notes, and probation officers. Several tools are provided to help the therapist and caregivers identify the extent of adolescent substance use.

- *Common Symptoms of Drug Use* (Handout 2.1) presents a list of symptoms that can be associated with substance use. The most salient symptoms are highlighted in boldface and pertain to associating with friends who are known drug users or at very high risk for substance abuse.
- Produced by NIDA, the *Commonly Abused Drugs Chart* (Handout 2.2) supplies information about drugs of abuse, their commercial and street names, routes of administration, intoxication effects, and potential health consequences. Therapists might find it helpful to have this chart in hand when completing the *Substance Use Chart* (Form 2.3) with youth. A website link to the *Commonly Abused Drugs Chart* (Handout 2.2) can be found, along with other helpful information, on the NIDA website (*www.nida.nih.gov/drugpages.html*; follow the link for *Commonly Abused Drugs Chart* or go directly to *www.nida.nih.gov/DrugPages/DrugsofAbuse.html*).
- The *Substance Use Chart* (Form 2.3) is a resource for obtaining and organizing drug use information that is used by several service provider agencies within the

South Carolina substance abuse treatment system. This tool can be used by therapists to record a complete history of substance use.

- As detailed in Chapter 7, valid measures of drug and alcohol use can be obtained relatively easily through urine drug screens and alcohol breath scans. These indices of substance use are extremely valuable in supplementing information obtained by self-report methods.

Determine the Impact of Substance Use and Possible Need for Treatment.

Assuming it has been determined that the youth is using drugs or alcohol, the next task for the therapist is to differentiate between experimental substance use, which is common for many youth during adolescence, and problematic substance use, which usually indicates a need for treatment. Screening tools can be used to help determine whether a particular youth has a substance use problem, and two of the most efficient are described and provided here.

- The *CAGE Questionnaire* (Mayfield, McLead, & Hall, 1974) is easy to use, and its four items can be asked by interview or in a paper-and-pencil questionnaire format. Therapists should also ask caregivers to respond to the CAGE questions concerning the youth. A "yes" response to any of the CAGE questions by either the youth or the caregiver indicates an increased likelihood that the adolescent's substance use is problematic. A *Modified CAGE Questionnaire* (Form 2.1) is provided to facilitate this assessment process.
- The *Client Substance Index—Short Form* (Form 2.2; Thomas, 1990) is another useful screening tool with 15 yes—no questions for the youth to complete. A "yes" response to any of the questions indicates that the youth's substance use warrants serious consideration as indicative of abuse or dependence.

Even when a youth has been referred specifically for substance use treatment, and the youth and caregiver already acknowledge that treatment is needed, therapists should still assess the extent to which drug use is ongoing and problematic. The impact of the drug use on the youth's functioning should be assessed in key domains of life—at home, in school, with peers, and in the broader community. The *Domains of Functioning* worksheet (Form 2.4) is provided to assist with this purpose. Although it might be apparent to the therapist that drug use is illegal and, therefore, puts the youth at risk, it is usually very helpful to talk about the linkages the therapist finds between drug and alcohol use and functional impairments the youth and family members might be experiencing (i.e., poor grades, arrests, probation, family arguments). Again, the general rule for deciding whether interventions for substance use are needed is based on an observed link between substance use and negative life outcomes or high risk for such outcomes.

If the therapist establishes a link between the youth's substance use and negative life outcomes, the next step is to ascertain the youth's and caregiver's appreciation of that link. Engaging an individual in treatment is easier when he or she sees a clear connection between the presenting problems, or what resulted in referral to therapy, and the intervention the therapist is seeking to implement. At this point in the assessment, the therapist will want to revisit youth and caregiver treatment goals (i.e., getting off probation, finding a job, improved school performance) and demonstrate how these goals can be better reached if the youth and family participate in substance abuse treatment. The most common challenge faced by the therapist attempting to engage families in substance abuse treatment is one in which the youth or the caregiver will not acknowledge that the youth has a substance abuse problem. Steps for addressing this challenge are outlined in the Troubleshooting Tips section of this chapter. The reader is encouraged to review the Family Engagement section in Chapter 3 for suggestions concerning how to address other engagement challenges that frequently arise during the assessment and early intervention process.

TROUBLESHOOTING TIPS

Objective

The purpose of this section is to help therapists anticipate common challenges to obtaining youth and caregiver participation in the *Determining the Need for Substance Use Treatment* component of CM and to suggest strategies to address these difficulties.

Challenges and Solutions

Neither Youth nor Caregiver Acknowledges Drug Problem.

If both the youth and the caregiver deny that the youth uses drugs when evidence suggests she or he is using drugs, or if they deny that such drug use is problematic when the therapist believes otherwise, the therapist should not attempt to implement the CM protocol. Instead, we recommend using drug screens for 4 to 6 weeks to gather evidence that the youth is or is not using drugs. If the drug screens are "clean" throughout this time, meaning no drugs are detected, then the drug screening procedures should be suspended. On the other hand, if the screens are "dirty," the inconsistency between the drug results and the clients' contentions should be addressed clinically. Likewise, the therapist should stay attuned to evidence that the youth's drug use is associated with problems in his or her life.

Youth Denies Drug Problem but Caregiver Acknowledges Drug Problem.

This is a common scenario. Assuming that the caregiver wishes to address the problem in spite of the adolescent's denial, we recommend that the therapist and the caregiver implement CM with the youth. If the adolescent is not having a problem with drug use, the screens will be clean and he or she will earn rewards. On the other hand, if the adolescent is having a problem with drug use, an appropriate intervention will be in place.

Youth Is Reluctant to Reveal Information to His or Her Caregiver.

The CM program presented in this manual strongly relies on caregiver involvement. Thus, therapists are encouraged to be creative in working with youth to secure their consent to involve their caregivers in treatment. Yet, given the concerns adolescents might have about revealing substance use information to their caregivers at the onset of treatment, it might make sense to conduct one or two of the early assessment sessions alone with the youth. To avoid subsequent problems in sharing adolescent drug use information with caregivers, however, therapists must obtain a signed consent from the youth allowing disclosure to caregivers. Therapists might want to use a one-to-one assessment session to help the adolescent determine how he or she would like to tell the caregiver about the drug use. It often helps if therapists find out what factors are driving the youth's difficulty in sharing information with the caregiver (i.e., shame, fear of consequences, concern about caregiver's feelings or reaction) and try to address these with the youth and caregiver prior to putting them in a session together.

A Note about Confidentiality. When a diagnosis of alcohol or drug abuse or dependency is made for the purpose of substance abuse treatment or referral for treatment, the client is protected under the federal confidentiality law 42 C. F. R Part 2. Additionally, all clients are protected under the Health Insurance Portability and Accountability Act (HIPAA). Both HIPAA and 42 C.F.R Part 2 protect minors as well as adults from unconsented disclosures in most situations. Thus, therapists generally cannot disclose information even to parents without the minor's consent. Clinicians are advised to become familiar with these two federal laws as well as the laws pertaining to confidentiality and disclosure specific to their state.

THERAPIST CHECKLIST, FORMS, AND HANDOUTS FOR CHAPTER 2: DETERMINING THE NEED FOR SUBSTANCE USE TREATMENT

THERAPIST FLOWCHART AND CHECKLIST 2.1

Determining the Need for Substance Use Treatment

Case number: ______________ **Session date:** ______________

Clarify presenting problems

Drug use is a presenting problem

Drug use is NOT a presenting problem

Determine if drug use problems might be present

___ Drug and alcohol use problems are often found in youth who present to clinics with other problems.

___ Therefore, I would like for us to work together to try and determine if (*youth's name*) might be using drugs or alcohol. Once we know if this is happening, we can then see if the drug use is causing problems that suggest she/he needs further treatment.

___ I would like to find out more from both of you about whether (*youth's name*) has had problems related to drug or alcohol use either recently or in the past. I am interested in knowing about any problems he/she may have had at home, in school, with friends, or with the law that might have involved drug or alcohol use.

___ [If clinically helpful, review a copy of *Common Symptoms of Drug Use* (Handout 2.1) with the caregiver and youth to elicit more information.]

___ [Remember to consider your experience with the youth, the caregiver's experience with the youth, how treatment is progressing, and information gathered from other informants (i.e., teachers, probation officer).]

Drug use concerns exist

Gather information on youth's drug use and severity of use

[CONTINUED ON NEXT PAGE]

Drug use problems are not elicited

___ [If substance use problems or potential problems are not elicited, but caregiver or therapist continues to have concerns, consider collecting random urine drug screens or alcohol breath scans to further determine if problems are present.]

[STOP]

[CONTINUED FROM PREVIOUS PAGE]

Drug use concerns exist

↓

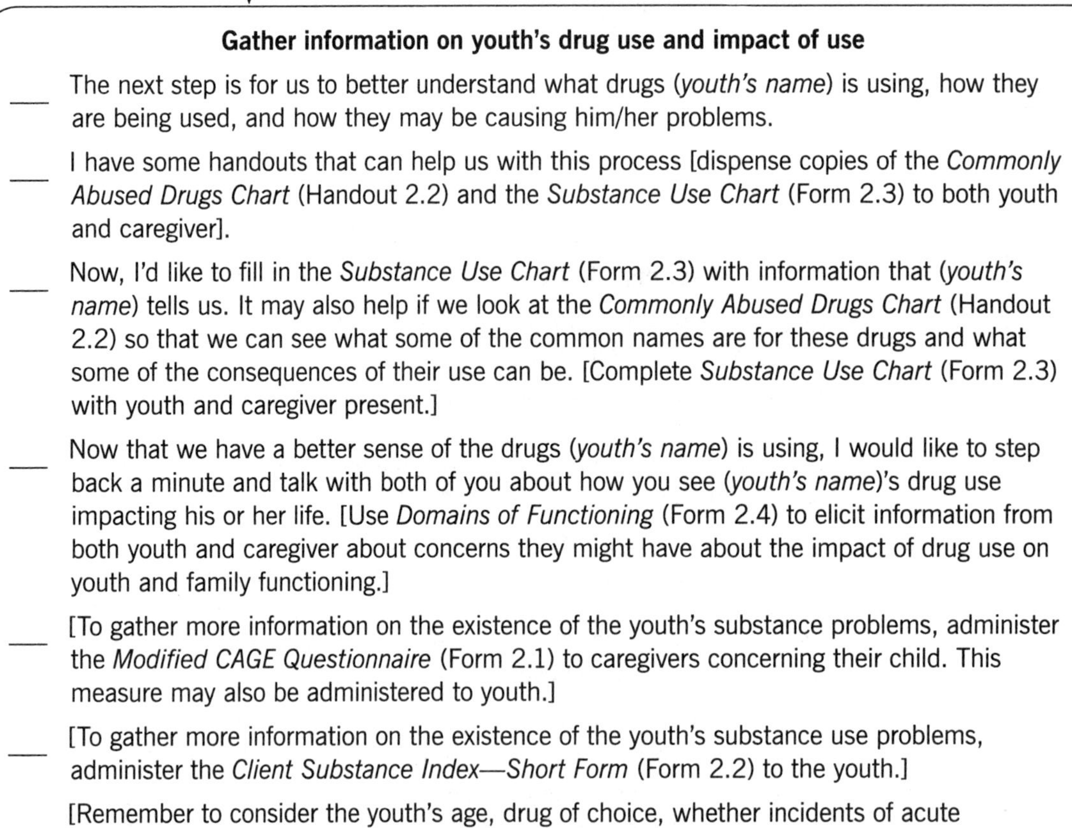

Gather information on youth's drug use and impact of use

___ The next step is for us to better understand what drugs (*youth's name*) is using, how they are being used, and how they may be causing him/her problems.

___ I have some handouts that can help us with this process [dispense copies of the *Commonly Abused Drugs Chart* (Handout 2.2) and the *Substance Use Chart* (Form 2.3) to both youth and caregiver].

___ Now, I'd like to fill in the *Substance Use Chart* (Form 2.3) with information that (*youth's name*) tells us. It may also help if we look at the *Commonly Abused Drugs Chart* (Handout 2.2) so that we can see what some of the common names are for these drugs and what some of the consequences of their use can be. [Complete *Substance Use Chart* (Form 2.3) with youth and caregiver present.]

___ Now that we have a better sense of the drugs (*youth's name*) is using, I would like to step back a minute and talk with both of you about how you see (*youth's name*)'s drug use impacting his or her life. [Use *Domains of Functioning* (Form 2.4) to elicit information from both youth and caregiver about concerns they might have about the impact of drug use on youth and family functioning.]

___ [To gather more information on the existence of the youth's substance problems, administer the *Modified CAGE Questionnaire* (Form 2.1) to caregivers concerning their child. This measure may also be administered to youth.]

___ [To gather more information on the existence of the youth's substance use problems, administer the *Client Substance Index—Short Form* (Form 2.2) to the youth.]

___ [Remember to consider the youth's age, drug of choice, whether incidents of acute ingestion of large quantities of the substances have occurred, and if drug use takes place in inappropriate settings (e.g., school).]

Substance use problems identified and linked to youth functional impairment

Caregiver and youth willing to engage in treatment

___ [Go to Chapter 3—Therapist Task 3.1: Introducing CM to Families.]

Caregiver or youth NOT willing to engage in treatment

___ [Go to Troubleshooting Tips section in this chapter and Family Engagement section in Chapter 3.]

Substance use NOT linked to youth functional impairment based on therapist and family opinion

___ Substance use interventions are not indicated at this time. Consider continuing to assess or collect information (i.e., random drug screens) about potential use and its impact on functioning.

[STOP]

FORM 2.1

Modified CAGE Questionnaire

QUESTIONS FOR YOUTH

1. Have you ever felt you ought to cut down on drinking or drug use? .... Y / N
2. Have people annoyed you by criticizing your drinking or drug use? .... Y / N
3. Have you ever felt bad or guilty about your drinking or drug use? .... Y / N
4. Have you ever had a drink or used drugs first thing in the morning .... Y / N
   to steady your nerves or get rid of a hangover?

QUESTIONS FOR CAREGIVER

1. Have you ever felt your child ought to cut down on drinking or drug use? .... Y / N
2. Have you and other people annoyed your child by criticizing his/her drinking .... Y / N
   or drug use?
3. Has your child ever felt bad or guilty about his/her drinking or drug use? .... Y / N
4. Has your child ever had a drink or used drugs first thing in the morning .... Y / N
   to steady his/her nerves or get rid of a hangover?

FORM 2.2

Client Substance Index—Short Form

Please read carefully and circle the appropriate response.

1. Have you ever done something crazy while high and had to make excuses for your behavior later? .... Y / N
2. Have you ever felt really burnt out for a day after using drugs? .... Y / N
3. Have you ever gotten out of bed in the morning and really felt wasted? .... Y / N
4. Did you ever get high in school? .... Y / N
5. Have you gotten into a fight while you were high, including drinking? .... Y / N
6. Do you think about getting high a lot of the time? .... Y / N
7. Have you ever thought about committing suicide when you were high? .... Y / N
8. Have you run away from home, partly because of an argument over drug use? .... Y / N
9. Did you ever try to stick to one drug after a bad experience mixing drugs? .... Y / N
10. Have you gotten into a physical fight during a family argument over drugs? .... Y / N
11. Have you ever been suspended because of something you did while high? .... Y / N
12. Have you ever had a beer or some booze to get over a hangover? .... Y / N
13. Do you usually keep a supply of drugs for emergencies, no matter how small? .... Y / N
14. Have you ever smoked some pot to get over a hangover? .... Y / N
15. Have you ever felt nervous or cranky after you stopped using for a while? .... Y / N

The Client Substance Index—Short Form was developed and evaluated as part of a larger Substance Abuse Screening protocol through the National Center for Juvenile Justice. From Thomas (1990).

FORM 2.3

Substance Use Chart

Interview the client to fully complete the grid.

Psychoactive Substance Use History					
Drug[a]	Age at first use	Frequency of use over past 12 months	Typical quantity of use	Date of last use	Route of use[b]
Alcohol					
Amphetamine					
Caffeine					
Cannabis					
Cocaine					
Hallucinogen					
Inhalant					
Nicotine					
Opioid					
PCP					
Sedative–hypnotic					
Other					

[a]Use the Commonly Abused Drugs Chart (Handout 2.2) for assistance in identifying examples for each drug category and slang words, as the youth might not always know the formal drug names.

[b]For example, smoked, ingested, injected, inhaled through nose, or absorbed via skin patch.

FORM 2.4

Domains of Functioning

HOME

1. How is the youth's communication with parents, siblings, and other family members? (Example: cooperative, quiet, withdrawn, moody, angry, agitated, defiant)

2. Does the youth fulfill responsibilities at home and follow family rules? (Example: chores, homework, routines, curfew, use of profanity)

(cont.)

3. How are responsibilities completed at home? (Example: well, on time, incompletely, avoids or refuses)

SCHOOL

4. How are the youth's grades in each subject in school? (Example: improving, stable, deteriorating, incomplete)

5. How is the youth's behavior in school? (Example: generally minds and is compliant, argumentative, gets suspensions or expulsions, on time, tardy, skipping class, truant from school)

(cont.)

PEERS

6. How would the youth's peers be described? Name key peers and their qualities. (Example: does peer attend school, have a job, obey the law, get arrested, use drugs, have problems in school or community?)

7. How is the youth's relationship with peers? (Example: positive, supportive, distant, argumentative, fighting; leader, follower)

COMMUNITY

8. How is the youth's behavior in the community? (Example: participates in sports, clubs, positive activities; has few activities, has problems with the law, formal legal charges, on probation)

HANDOUT 2.1

Common Symptoms of Drug Use

Things others might see:

- ***Friends who use drugs or have problems in school***
- ***Friends who have been arrested***
- ***Older friends who are not working or going to school***
- Rapid or unusual changes in mood
- Poor coordination
- Slowed or rapid speech
- Inability to remember recent events
- Fast or slowed behavior and reaction times
- Changes in appetite
- Sleepiness
- Apathy
- Being silly for no reason
- Bloodshot eyes
- Poor sports performance
- Poor school performance
- Lingering odors of marijuana or attempts to cover up odors
- Clothing or property that promotes drug use

Things the youth might report (in addition to the above symptoms):

- ***Hanging out with friends who use drugs or do poorly in school***
- ***Hanging out with friends who get in trouble with the law***
- ***Hanging out with older friends who are not working or going to school***
- Racing or slowed thoughts
- Racing heart rate (stimulants, cocaine)
- Unusual thoughts or paranoid beliefs
- Feeling disconnected from reality
- Lack of motivation

Bold italics denote important clinical factors that are frequently linked with youth drug use and relapse.

HANDOUT 2.2

NIDA NATIONAL INSTITUTE ON DRUG ABUSE

Commonly Abused Drugs

Visit NIDA at www.drugabuse.gov

National Institutes of Health
U.S. Department of Health and Human Services

Substances: Category and Name	Examples of *Commercial* and Street Names	DEA Schedule*/ How Administered**	*Acute Effects*/Health Risks
Tobacco			*Increased blood pressure and heart rate*/chronic lung disease; cardiovascular disease; stroke; cancers of the mouth, pharynx, larynx, esophagus, stomach, pancreas, cervix, kidney, bladder, and acute myeloid leukemia; adverse pregnancy outcomes; addiction
Nicotine	Found in cigarettes, cigars, bidis, and smokeless tobacco (snuff, spit tobacco, chew)	Not scheduled/smoked, snorted, chewed	
Alcohol			*In low doses, euphoria, mild stimulation, relaxation, lowered inhibitions; in higher doses, drowsiness, slurred speech, nausea, emotional volatility, loss of coordination, visual distortions, impaired memory, sexual dysfunction, loss of consciousness*/increased risk of injuries, violence, fetal damage (in pregnant women); depression; neurologic deficits; hypertension; liver and heart disease; addiction; fatal overdose
Alcohol (ethyl alcohol)	Found in liquor, beer, and wine	Not scheduled/swallowed	
Cannabinoids			*Euphoria; relaxation; slowed reaction time; distorted sensory perception; impaired balance and coordination; increased heart rate and appetite; impaired learning, memory; anxiety; panic attacks; psychosis*/cough; frequent respiratory infections; possible mental health decline; addiction
Marijuana	Blunt, dope, ganja, grass, herb, joint, bud, Mary Jane, pot, reefer, green, trees, smoke, sinsemilla, skunk, weed	I/smoked, swallowed	
Hashish	Boom, gangster, hash, hash oil, hemp	I/smoked, swallowed	
Opioids			*Euphoria; drowsiness; impaired coordination; dizziness; confusion; nausea; sedation; feeling of heaviness in the body; slowed or arrested breathing*/constipation; endocarditis; hepatitis; HIV; addiction; fatal overdose
Heroin	*Diacetylmorphine:* smack, horse, brown sugar, dope, H, junk, skag, skunk, white horse, China white; cheese (with OTC cold medicine and antihistamine)	I/injected, smoked, snorted	
Opium	*Laudanum, paregoric:* big O, black stuff, block, gum, hop	II, III, V/swallowed, smoked	
Stimulants			*Increased heart rate, blood pressure, body temperature, metabolism; feelings of exhilaration; increased energy, mental alertness; tremors; reduced appetite; irritability; anxiety; panic; paranoia; violent behavior; psychosis*/weight loss; insomnia; cardiac or cardiovascular complications; stroke; seizures; addiction **Also, for cocaine**—nasal damage from snorting **Also, for methamphetamine**—severe dental problems
Cocaine	*Cocaine hydrochloride:* blow, bump, C, candy, Charlie, coke, crack, flake, rock, snow, toot	II/snorted, smoked, injected	
Amphetamine	*Biphetamine, Dexedrine:* bennies, black beauties, crosses, hearts, LA turnaround, speed, truck drivers, uppers	II/swallowed, snorted, smoked, injected	
Methamphetamine	*Desoxyn:* meth, ice, crank, chalk, crystal, fire, glass, go fast, speed	II/swallowed, snorted, smoked, injected	
Club Drugs			***MDMA**—mild hallucinogenic effects; increased tactile sensitivity, empathic feelings; lowered inhibition; anxiety; chills; sweating; teeth clenching; muscle cramping/*sleep disturbances; depression; impaired memory; hyperthermia; addiction **Flunitrazepam**—*sedation; muscle relaxation; confusion; memory loss; dizziness; impaired coordination*/addiction **GHB**—*drowsiness; nausea; headache; disorientation; loss of coordination; memory loss*/unconsciousness; seizures; coma
MDMA (methylenedioxymethamphetamine)	Ecstasy, Adam, clarity, Eve, lover's speed, peace, uppers	I/swallowed, snorted, injected	
Flunitrazepam***	*Rohypnol:* forget-me pill, Mexican Valium, R2, roach, Roche, roofies, roofinol, rope, rophies	IV/swallowed, snorted	
GHB***	*Gamma-hydroxybutyrate:* G, Georgia home boy, grievous bodily harm, liquid ecstasy, soap, scoop, goop, liquid X	I/swallowed	
Dissociative Drugs			*Feelings of being separate from one's body and environment; impaired motor function*/anxiety; tremors; numbness; memory loss; nausea **Also, for ketamine**—*analgesia; impaired memory; delirium; respiratory depression and arrest; death* **Also, for PCP and analogs**—*analgesia; psychosis; aggression; violence; slurred speech; loss of coordination; hallucinations* **Also, for DXM**—*euphoria; slurred speech; confusion; dizziness; distorted visual perceptions*
Ketamine	*Ketalar SV:* cat Valium, K, Special K, vitamin K	III/injected, snorted, smoked	
PCP and analogs	*Phencyclidine:* angel dust, boat, hog, love boat, peace pill	I, II/swallowed, smoked, injected	
Salvia divinorum	Salvia, Shepherdess's Herb, Maria Pastora, magic mint, Sally-D	Not scheduled/chewed, swallowed, smoked	
Dextromethorphan (DXM)	Found in some cough and cold medications: Robotripping, Robo, Triple C	Not scheduled/swallowed	
Hallucinogens			*Altered states of perception and feeling; hallucinations; nausea* **Also, for LSD and mescaline**—*increased body temperature, heart rate, blood pressure; loss of appetite; sweating; sleeplessness; numbness; dizziness; weakness; tremors; impulsive behavior; rapid shifts in emotion* **Also, for LSD**—Flashbacks, Hallucinogen Persisting Perception Disorder **Also, for psilocybin**—*nervousness; paranoia; panic*
LSD	*Lysergic acid diethylamide:* acid, blotter, cubes, microdot, yellow sunshine, blue heaven	I/swallowed, absorbed through mouth tissues	
Mescaline	Buttons, cactus, mesc, peyote	I/swallowed, smoked	
Psilocybin	Magic mushrooms, purple passion, shrooms, little smoke	I/swallowed	
Other Compounds			**Steroids**—*no intoxication effects*/hypertension; blood clotting and cholesterol changes; liver cysts; hostility and aggression; acne; in adolescents—premature stoppage of growth; in males—prostate cancer, reduced sperm production, shrunken testicles, breast enlargement; in females—menstrual irregularities, development of beard and other masculine characteristics **Inhalants** *(varies by chemical)—stimulation; loss of inhibition; headache; nausea or vomiting; slurred speech; loss of motor coordination; wheezing*/cramps; muscle weakness; depression; memory impairment; damage to cardiovascular and nervous systems; unconsciousness; sudden death
Anabolic steroids	*Anadrol, Oxandrin, Durabolin, Depo-Testosterone, Equipoise:* roids, juice, gym candy, pumpers	III/injected, swallowed, applied to skin	
Inhalants	*Solvents (paint thinners, gasoline, glues); gases (butane, propane, aerosol propellants, nitrous oxide); nitrites (isoamyl, isobutyl, cyclohexyl):* laughing gas, poppers, snappers, whippets	Not scheduled/inhaled through nose or mouth	

(cont.)

Substances: Category and Name	Examples of *Commercial* and Street Names	DEA Schedule*/ How Administered**	*Acute Effects*/Health Risks
Prescription Medications			
CNS Depressants Stimulants Opioid Pain Relievers	For more information on prescription medications, please visit http://www.nida.nih.gov/DrugPages/PrescripDrugsChart.html.		

** Schedule I and II drugs have a high potential for abuse. They require greater storage security and have a quota on manufacturing, among other restrictions. Schedule I drugs are available for research only and have no approved medical use; Schedule II drugs are available only by prescription (unrefillable) and require a form for ordering. Schedule III and IV drugs are available by prescription, may have five refills in 6 months, and may be ordered orally. Some Schedule V drugs are available over the counter.*

*** Some of the health risks are directly related to the route of drug administration. For example, injection drug use can increase the risk of infection through needle contamination with staphylococci, HIV, hepatitis, and other organisms.*

**** Associated with sexual assaults.*

Principles of Drug Addiction Treatment

More than three decades of scientific research show that treatment can help drug-addicted individuals stop drug use, avoid relapse and successfully recover their lives. Based on this research, 13 fundamental principles that characterize effective drug abuse treatment have been developed. These principles are detailed in *NIDA's Principles of Drug Addiction Treatment: A Research-Based Guide.* The guide also describes different types of science-based treatments and provides answers to commonly asked questions.

1. **Addiction is a complex but treatable disease that affects brain function and behavior.** Drugs alter the brain's structure and how it functions, resulting in changes that persist long after drug use has ceased. This may help explain why abusers are at risk for relapse even after long periods of abstinence.
2. **No single treatment is appropriate for everyone.** Matching treatment settings, interventions, and services to an individual's particular problems and needs is critical to his or her ultimate success.
3. **Treatment needs to be readily available.** Because drug-addicted individuals may be uncertain about entering treatment, taking advantage of available services the moment people are ready for treatment is critical. Potential patients can be lost if treatment is not immediately available or readily accessible.
4. **Effective treatment attends to multiple needs of the individual, not just his or her drug abuse.** To be effective, treatment must address the individual's drug abuse and any associated medical, psychological, social, vocational, and legal problems.
5. **Remaining in treatment for an adequate period of time is critical.** The appropriate duration for an individual depends on the type and degree of his or her problems and needs. Research indicates that most addicted individuals need at least 3 months in treatment to significantly reduce or stop their drug use and that the best outcomes occur with longer durations of treatment.
6. **Counseling—individual and/or group—and other behavioral therapies are the most commonly used forms of drug abuse treatment.** Behavioral therapies vary in their focus and may involve addressing a patient's motivations to change, building skills to resist drug use, replacing drug-using activities with constructive and rewarding activities, improving problemsolving skills, and facilitating better interpersonal relationships.
7. **Medications are an important element of treatment for many patients, especially when combined with counseling and other behavioral therapies.** For example, methadone and buprenorphine are effective in helping individuals addicted to heroin or other opioids stabilize their lives and reduce their illicit drug use. Also, for persons addicted to nicotine, a nicotine replacement product (nicotine patches or gum) or an oral medication (buproprion or varenicline), can be an effective component of treatment when part of a comprehensive behavioral treatment program.
8. **An individual's treatment and services plan must be assessed continually and modified as necessary to ensure it meets his or her changing needs.** A patient may require varying combinations of services and treatment components during the course of treatment and recovery. In addition to counseling or psychotherapy, a patient may require medication, medical services, family therapy, parenting instruction, vocational rehabilitation and/or social and legal services. For many patients, a continuing care approach provides the best results, with treatment intensity varying according to a person's changing needs.
9. **Many drug-addicted individuals also have other mental disorders.** Because drug abuse and addiction—both of which are mental disorders—often co-occur with other mental illnesses, patients presenting with one condition should be assessed for the other(s). And when these problems co-occur, treatment should address both (or all), including the use of medications as appropriate.
10. **Medically assisted detoxification is only the first stage of addiction treatment and by itself does little to change long-term drug abuse.** Although medically assisted detoxification can safely manage the acute physical symptoms of withdrawal, detoxification alone is rarely sufficient to help addicted individuals achieve long-term abstinence. Thus, patients should be encouraged to continue drug treatment following detoxification.
11. **Treatment does not need to be voluntary to be effective.** Sanctions or enticements from family, employment settings, and/or the criminal justice system can significantly increase treatment entry, retention rates, and the ultimate success of drug treatment interventions.
12. **Drug use during treatment must be monitored continuously, as lapses during treatment do occur.** Knowing their drug use is being monitored can be a powerful incentive for patients and can help them withstand urges to use drugs. Monitoring also provides an early indication of a return to drug use, signaling a possible need to adjust an individual's treatment plan to better meet his or her needs.
13. **Treatment programs should assess patients for the presence of HIV/AIDS, hepatitis B and C, tuberculosis, and other infectious diseases, as well as provide targeted risk-reduction counseling to help patients modify or change behaviors that place them at risk of contracting or spreading infectious diseases.** Targeted counseling specifically focused on reducing infectious disease risk can help patients further reduce or avoid substance-related and other high-risk behaviors. Treatment providers should encourage and support HIV screening and inform patients that highly active antiretroviral therapy (HAART) has proven effective in combating HIV, including among drug-abusing populations.

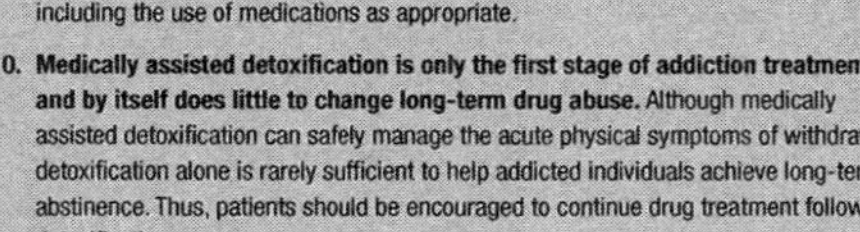

This chart may be reprinted. Citation of the source is appreciated.

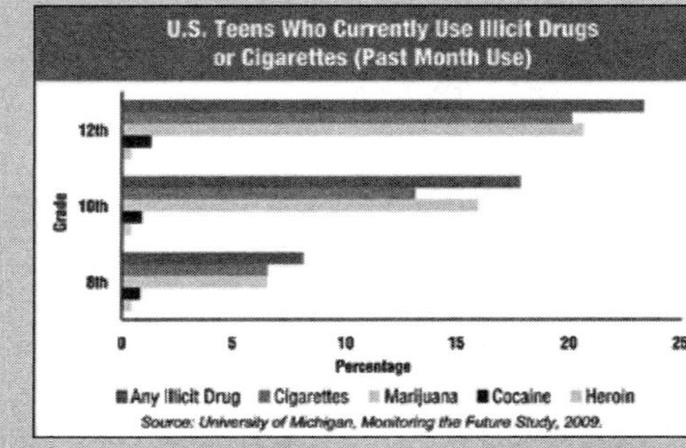

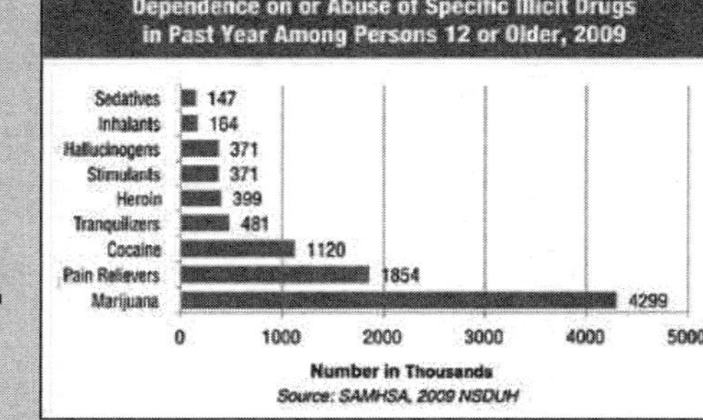

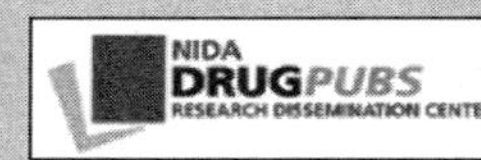

Order NIDA publications from DrugPubs:
1-877-643-2644 or 1-240-645-0228 (TTY/TDD)

Revised October 2010

Sample Dialogue: Determining the Need for Substance Use Treatment

INTRODUCTION TO TONY AND HIS MOTHER, MS. SMITH

Tony, a 16-year-old Caucasian male, was referred to the clinic by the Department of Juvenile Justice because he was arrested for possession of a small amount of marijuana. His records indicate that he has a history of truancy and has been suspended from school once this year for fighting. He risks expulsion from school if further problems occur. At intake, Tony denied symptoms of anxiety, depression, posttraumatic stress disorder, mania, or psychosis as well as current or past suicidal or homicidal ideation. Tony lives with his mother and stepfather in an apartment situated in a working-class neighborhood. His mother works as an administrative assistant and his stepfather is a mechanic. Tony has not seen his biological father in 10 years.

The therapist met with Tony and his mother, Ms. Smith, the week prior to complete the necessary intake paperwork and obtain consents for treatment. During that session the caregiver endorsed Items 1 and 2 of the caregiver section of the *Modified CAGE Questionnaire* (Form 2.1) as a concern and Tony endorsed Items 5 and 11 of the *Client Substance Index—Short Form* (Form 2.2), indicating that he had gotten into a fight while high and was subsequently suspended from school for that behavior. On the *Domains of Functioning* (Form 2.4) Tony's mother described some history of antisocial behavior, including minor theft and fighting in a group. She stated that Tony enjoys playing basketball and does well in history class. He is functioning at grade level in all subjects except math and is getting C's in most classes. Tony has a few close friends who also use drugs and a girlfriend whom the mother believes gets good grades and does not use drugs.

This week the therapist is meeting with the family to try and better understand their presenting problems and goals for treatment.

CLARIFY PRESENTING PROBLEMS

Therapist: Hi, welcome back. It is good to see you again.

Caregiver: Thank you, good to see you too.

Therapist: Tony, why don't you sit down over here, where we can see you better?

Tony: I don't see why I need to be here. I'm gonna just sit here. How long til we're done?

Therapist: Okay, your mom and I can just pull our chairs to you. Sounds like you would prefer not to be here.

Tony: You got that right.

Caregiver: Tony, you better show some respect!

Therapist: It's okay, Ms. Smith. That is a very normal response. It takes most of the young men I work with a little while to get used to treatment.

Tony: Treatment? I don't need treatment! What kind of place is this?

Therapist: This is a clinic where we help young people who are having problems of some kind.

Tony: I don't have any problems, except that my mom made me come here. That is my only problem.

Therapist: Ms. Smith, can you tell me more about what has brought you here?

Caregiver: Well, like I told you last week, Tony got caught with a bag of pot by a policeman about a month ago. He was arrested and put on probation.

Tony: It wasn't my stuff. I was just holding it for somebody.

Caregiver: Please, Tony, I know you have been using and I also know that the probation officer keeps getting dirty screens on you. That is why we are here. You are going to get in trouble if you don't get clean.

Tony: That PO is just bluffing. He likes to scare people.

Caregiver: Well, I am afraid he might lock you away.

Tony: Maybe, but at least then I wouldn't have to go to school.

Therapist: So, Ms. Smith, it sounds like you are here because you would like for Tony to stay out of prison.

Caregiver: Right.

Therapist: Are you worried about Tony using? Do you want him to get off drugs?

Caregiver: Of course! I want him to quit. I would want him to quit even if he had not been arrested.

Therapist: Okay, good. One of the first things I like to do is find out why a family has come to me. It helps if I understand what each person wants to get out of treatment, what their goals are.

Tony: Well, my goal is to get out of here.

Therapist: All right, so getting released from treatment is your goal.

Tony: I guess.

Therapist: What do you think it will take to be released from treatment?

Tony: I don't know.

Caregiver: Oh please, you know you have to get clean. This therapist has to tell your PO you are participating or you may end up in prison.

Tony: Okay, I guess my goal is to get off probation. So my goal is to get clean so I can get off probation.

Therapist: Do you have any other goals?

Tony: What do you mean?

Therapist: Well, lots of teens whom I help get off drugs also find that they do better in school and in sports once the drugs are out of their system. Do you think that getting off drugs might help you in any way?

Tony: Well, I like basketball. I'd like to be better at basketball, so I guess that's a goal.

Caregiver: Don't forget school, son. You used to get A's and B's; now you get C's.

Tony: I know, I don't like school, it's boring and stupid.

Therapist: Do you want to graduate?

Tony: Of course. I'm no dropout.

Caregiver: He better graduate.

Therapist: Do you know what you want to do when you grow up?

Tony: Play basketball, NBA.

Therapist: Wow, you have big aspirations. That would be wonderful. Something tells me you will really want to get off pot if you hope to play ball. Even high school basketball can be pretty strenuous.

Caregiver: He has other, more reasonable plans too. Tony, tell her what else you might want to do.

Tony: I have an uncle who owns some trucks. He told me that I can drive for him when I get older if I get my trucking license.

Therapist: That sounds like a good plan too. So, to summarize, I hear that you, Tony, have a number of good reasons to get off drugs. These reasons include not wanting to go to prison, wanting to get off probation, hoping to be in good physical health so that you can play basketball, and trying to get your license so that you can drive trucks one day.

Tony: Yeah, I guess that sums it up.

Therapist: Ms. Smith, you would like for Tony to get off probation, stay out of prison, go to school, and get a good job one day.

Caregiver: Yes, that is correct. I think Tony also needs to start thinking about his future more. He is already in the 10th grade. He will be grown up before he knows it.

Therapist: Right, hopefully as we help Tony get off drugs, we can also in effect be helping him to mature and grow up.

GATHER INFORMATION ON THE YOUTH'S DRUG USE AND IMPACT OF USE

Therapist: Now that we all seem to be in agreement that it makes sense for us to work together to help Tony get off drugs, I have a few more things I need to find out before we can get started in treatment.

Tony: Now what?

Therapist: Don't worry, it's not very hard. I just need to make sure that I understand what drugs you are using. I need to know what drugs you use to be able to help you stop using them. [Gives each participant a copy of *Substance Use Chart* (Form 2.3) and *Commonly Abused Drugs Chart* (Handout 2.2).] All right, now I would like to use this chart [Form 2.3] to help me assess the drugs you may have used in the past as well as the ones you are using now.

Tony: I told you, I only use pot.

Therapist: Okay, let's start there. The technical term for pot is cannabis. How old were you the first time you tried pot?

Tony: Do I have to tell you this? My mom is sitting right here.

Therapist: Does that bother you?

Tony: Yeah, makes me feel weird. It's creepy talking about drugs in front of your mom.

Therapist: I know it takes a little while to get used to, but, yes, it is important that she be here.

Tony: Why?

Therapist: If your mom is not here with us, then she can't hear what we say and so she might miss out on important information that she needs to know in order to help you.

Tony: Can't you just tell her what I say?

Therapist: Well, I could try, but I might forget something, and it would not be a very efficient way to do this. It would take me twice as much time. I'm too busy to meet twice. Plus, I've found that doing it this way works better.

Caregiver: I'll try not to say anything. I'll just listen.

Therapist: That may help. I've found that after a few sessions, most teens get used to having their parents participate. It just takes a little while to adjust.

Tony: Whatever.

Therapist: So, let's get back to the form. Can you tell me how old you were when you first used?

Tony: I think I was 13, maybe 14.

Caregiver: What? Who were you with?

Tony: See what I mean? My mom is going to make me not want to say anything.

Caregiver: Sorry, I had no idea. I just feel like such a bad parent, and it makes me so mad.

Therapist: Those are all very normal feelings. Not to worry. The fact that you are here working on this shows me that you are a good, caring parent. It's hard for us to control all of the things that come into our kids' lives. So I'm glad you are able to step back and listen.

Tony: Okay, I was 13. That's all I'm going to say.

Therapist: That's enough about the past. Let's focus on the present. How much pot do you typically use in a day?

Tony: Well, some days I don't use any.

Therapist: Think about the last week. When did you last use?

Tony: Two days ago, on Saturday.

Therapist: Okay. Before that?

Tony: I think I used two other times last week, once on Wednesday, then again on Friday and Saturday.

Therapist: How much?

Tony: About one to two blunts, sometimes three each time.

Therapist: Did you share with anyone?

Tony: Yeah, each time I smoked the blunts with one or two, maybe three other people.

Therapist: Okay, let me fill that information in [*Substance Use Chart* (Form 2.3)].

Tony: What is this other paper for [*Commonly Abused Drugs Chart* (Handout 2.2)]?

Therapist: I like to use this sort of like a cheat sheet. It helps me remember the various street names of the drugs. That way, if one of the young adults I'm working with calls a drug something unusual, I can look it up.

Tony: Yeah, I've never seen the names of half these things either.

Therapist: Let's go down the list so I can find out what other drugs you may have tried.

Tony: I haven't done anything else on this list. [Holds up *Commonly Abused Drugs Chart* (Handout 2.2).]

Therapist: Please look at the other chart. How about that one [*Substance Use Chart* (Form 2.3)]?

Tony: Well, I tried cigarettes once, but hated it. They made me feel sick. Oh, and I drink caffeine sometimes.

Therapist: How much?

Tony: I dunno, I like energy drinks every once and awhile. But they cost too much.

Caregiver: He drinks iced tea and coffee sometimes. I'm more worried about alcohol. My brother has an alcohol problem, so I know it runs in my family. That really makes me worry.

Therapist: Tony, can you tell me about your alcohol use?

Tony: Well, I used some when I was younger.

Therapist: How young?

Tony: Thirteen, about the time I first had pot.

Therapist: When was the last time you drank?

Tony: Oh, a couple of months ago. I got tipsy at my friend's party. They were straight, didn't have any blunts, so I had to drink.

Therapist: How much did you drink?

Tony: Three or four beers.

Therapist: How about the time before last? When was that?

Tony: Can't remember. I think I average drinking about four, maybe five, times a year. Mostly on special occasions like holidays. I prefer pot.

Caregiver: That still concerns me.

Therapist: Tony, any idea why your mom is concerned?

Tony: Because she is afraid I will be a drunk like Uncle Henry.

Caregiver: I am also afraid you will drink and drive or drink and do something stupid like fight or steal.

Therapist: Those sound like valid concerns, mom. I noticed from the forms you both completed that Tony has been suspended from school for fighting while high. He has also been arrested for possessing marijuana and his grades have fallen from A's and B's to C's at school for the past 18 months. Are there other ways that either of you can think of that drugs are affecting Tony negatively?

Tony: I think you are exaggerating a little. It's not as bad as it sounds.

Caregiver: Can you believe that? He is in total denial.

Therapist: That is very normal and we will be looking at Tony's drug use so carefully in treatment that you won't have to worry about denial. Are there other ways that Tony's drug use is causing problems?

Caregiver: Yes, my husband and I fight more when Tony uses.

Therapist: Okay, good to know. I would like for your husband to come in sometime so that I can meet him. We can include him in some sessions.

Caregiver: I don't know if he can. He works long hours.

Therapist: Well, the door is always open for him to attend and I will be glad to talk to him on the phone sometime with you if you like.

Caregiver: Thanks, I'll keep that in mind.

Therapist: All right, let me stop us here for a minute so I can summarize what I have discovered so far.

Tony: Sure, go ahead.

Therapist: Tony primarily uses marijuana. As a therapist, I would say that marijuana is Tony's "drug of choice."

Tony: Yep.

Therapist: Tony's drug use is significant enough that it has caused him to get arrested and has contributed to declining grades, a school suspension, and disturbed relationships with his mother and stepfather.

Tony: Yep, screaming matches.

Therapist: Also, it seems that Tony uses alcohol from time to time and that use may also pose a threat to his well-being.

Caregiver: Right, so can we work on both alcohol and pot?

Therapist: One nice thing about the treatment I am going to provide is that we will be able to work on both things at the same time. So, while we will focus on marijuana, we will also test for alcohol and other drugs periodically. In other words, we will work together to help Tony get off both pot and alcohol. [Transitions into introducing contingency management, as outlined in Chapter 3.]

CHAPTER 3

Introducing Contingency Management and Engaging Families in Treatment

THERAPIST GOALS

1. **Introduce the CM program as an effective treatment for substance use.**
2. **Outlinc the four components of the CM program and estimate the length of treatment.**
3. **Engage the youth and caregivers in treatment and address potential barriers to engagement.**

The therapist sets the stage for CM implementation by noting the widespread effectiveness of CM in treating substance abuse and providing the youth and caregivers with a brief overview of the four major components of CM. Throughout all treatment sessions, the therapist maintains a positive, optimistic approach with the family, promotes family involvement, and addresses family engagement difficulties.

OVERVIEW OF CM

CM is a type of treatment that has been proven to help both adults and adolescents stop using drugs. It has been shown to help people who have alcohol or drug (marijuana, cocaine, and opium/heroin) dependence even when those problems have been long lasting. This type of treatment has four components and involves caregivers as well as the adolescent receiving treatment.

The Four Components of CM

The four components of CM are:

1. *The ABC assessment*—The therapist helps the youth and caregiver identify the people, places, feelings, thoughts, and situations that trigger the youth's use of drugs.
2. *Developing skills*—The therapist collaborates with the family to teach the youth skills for managing triggers of the drug use (*self-management planning, drug refusal skills training*) and helps him or her practice using and modifying these skills based on the results of drug screens.
3. *The point-and-level system with contract*—This part of CM involves developing and signing a contract for abstinence with the youth that outlines how urine screens and alcohol breath scans will be collected and what rewards can be earned in return for clean screens. The steps to this process include:
    a. *Identifying motivational rewards*—The youth, therapist, and caregiver develop a list of privileges and things that the youth would like to earn for clean drug screens and alcohol breath scans.
    b. *Personalizing the contract*—The therapist, caregiver, and the youth work together to describe in detail what privileges, activities, and items the youth can earn in return for having clean drug screens and alcohol breath scans.
    c. *Signing the contract*—The contract is signed and becomes a working agreement among the youth, caregiver, and therapist.
4. *Monitoring drug use*—Urine drug screens and alcohol breath scans are collected at least once a week to track the youth's progress. When screens and scans are clean, the youth earns the rewards specified in the contract.

Although the components of CM are described in a particular order in this book, therapists may choose to introduce them to families in a different order if clinically indicated. For instance, some therapists prefer to start treatment by having families sign the point-and-level system contract, while others prefer to start CM with urine drug screen collection. As therapists become more comfortable implementing CM, they might want to change the order in which the components are introduced to families.

Length of Treatment

The introduction to CM can be completed in about 30 minutes, and the subsequent orientations to the four components (Chapters 4–7) usually take 60 to 90 minutes each to complete, for a total of 4 to 6 hours of session time. Succeeding weekly therapy sessions will include all four components. That is, the therapist will *monitor substance use* by collecting a urine screen or having the caregiver report on the results of the screens for that week. The therapist will then ensure that the *point-and-level reward system contract* was followed, that points were added or taken away, and that rewards were given or withheld. Then the therapist, youth, and caregiver will complete an ABC assessment of the youth's substance use or nonuse that week. On the basis of the results of the ABC assessment, the therapist and family will modify the youth's *self-management plans* and *drug refusal skills* strategies as indicated. The length of CM treatment will vary depending on the youth's and family's response and involvement in treatment. The program can be usually completed in approximately 14 to 18 weeks.

FAMILY ENGAGEMENT

Throughout this book, a strong emphasis is placed on engaging caregivers in the treatment of their adolescent's substance abuse. This emphasis stems from two sets of important research findings noted in Chapter 1:

- Low caregiver supervision and inconsistent discipline are significant risk factors in adolescent substance abuse.
- Family involvement in treatment has been clearly linked with an increased probability of success with adolescent substance abusers.

Hence, the variation of CM described in this book involves caregivers in all clinical interventions and provides tips to help therapists bring caregivers into the treatment process. In those instances where, unfortunately, caregivers cannot be involved in treatment, suggestions are made for implementing CM in their absence (see Chapter 9).

In light of the critical role of caregivers in the implementation of CM with adolescents, therapists should plan on spending considerable time engaging the youth and family in treatment. Such engagement often requires considerable therapeutic skill, as caregivers frequently feel angry, tired, overwhelmed, and hopeless concerning their youth's substance use, and adolescents are often oppositional and uncooperative early in treatment. Thus, when thinking about laying the foundation for treatment, consider the following:

- Set the tone—CM is an intervention that is done *cooperatively* between therapist and family members. While the therapist has expert knowledge and skills to share, the family will be key participants in setting goals and implementing interventions.

- Get on the same page—the youth and caregivers play central roles in the clinical process. Therefore, the therapist must align with family members by showing that he or she understands each of their goals for treatment.

- Link youth and caregiver goals with the CM intervention—connecting the youth and caregiver's treatment goals with CM (i.e., helping the youth get off drugs) is important to facilitate engagement. For example, both youth and caregiver might want the adolescent to be more successful in school or to stay out of trouble with the law. The therapist can explain how CM can help achieve these goals by eliminating substance use.

- Maintain a supportive, yet firm, stance toward the youth—while the youth's drug use likely makes sense in some way, such behavior puts the youth at risk for many short- and long-term problems. The therapist models to the family acceptance of the youth's drug use without blaming or anger, while maintaining a firm stance that the youth is expected to get off drugs.

- Maintain a strength-focused approach with the youth and family. For example, do not emphasize those aspects of family functioning that might have contributed to the adolescent's substance abuse (e.g., poor monitoring, high conflict). Rather, stress strengths observed in the family (e.g., willingness to work on problems, love and concern for each other, sense of humor, social skills, employment, good grades).

In summary, youth are going to have the best chance of getting off of drugs when their caregivers are involved. The role of caregivers is very important as they are needed to help supervise, monitor, and set rules so that their children will learn to develop their own internal rules and good judgment over time. Caregivers are also needed to coach youth and help them develop the skills needed to get by in this very difficult, drug-filled world.

Aims and Time Frame of the Following Tasks

There are essentially two broad goals to accomplish at this stage in treatment. The first is to teach families about CM, its components, and proven effectiveness. The second is to assess the family's engagement in treatment and to address potential barriers that might arise. Therapists need anywhere from 20 minutes to a full hour to complete the tasks outlined in this chapter. The length of time needed varies substantially depending upon the family's level of engagement and their ease in comprehending and discussing the materials.

THERAPIST TASK 3.1: INTRODUCING CM TO FAMILIES

Objectives

1. Introduce the CM program as an effective treatment for substance use.
2. Outline the four components of the CM program.
3. Provide information about the length of treatment.

Material

- *Therapist Checklist 3.1: Introducing Contingency Management*

Accomplishing the Objectives

The importance of maintaining a hopeful and optimistic stance cannot be overemphasized. The next section of this chapter considers some of the keys to engendering hope, and these are pertinent throughout the entire course of treatment. For present purposes, as presented in *Therapist Checklist 3.1: Introducing Contingency Management*, the therapist begins by noting the general effectiveness of CM in reducing the use of substances such as marijuana, cocaine, and alcohol. Then the therapist emphasizes the importance of the youth and caregivers working together throughout treatment, and briefly describes the key components of CM (i.e., ABC assessment, monitoring drug use, point-and-level system with contract, and developing self-management and drug refusal skill.). Finally, the practitioner provides an estimated time frame for the duration of treatment, which is in the 14- to 18-week range.

THERAPIST TASK 3.2: ENGAGING THE FAMILY IN TREATMENT

Objectives

1. Ensure that treatment is a collaboration between the therapist and family.
2. Make sure that family members and the therapist are on the same page regarding both treatment goals and methods to achieve them.
3. Stay positive and strength focused.
4. Model firm but accepting and well-reasoned behavior for the caregivers.

Material

- *Therapist Checklist 3.2: Engaging the Family in Treatment*

Accomplishing the Objectives

In contrast with the emphases of most of this treatment manual, engaging families in treatment is more of a process and less subject to well-specified protocols. Consequently, this section and *Therapist Checklist 3.2: Engaging the Family in Treatment* are intended as frequent reminders of the styles of therapeutic communications that are valuable in successfully engaging families in treatment and are applicable to every session held with the youth and family. Overall, engagement processes emphasize the importance of collaboration and the development of mutual agreement on treatment goals and methods to achieve these goals. Therapist characteristics such as warmth and empathy are critical to obtaining such collaboration, and specific behaviors that recognize the strengths and efforts of family members will facilitate engagement as well. Although youth and caregivers might present many challenges to the implementation of CM, therapists should not waver from maintaining a positive and hopeful approach with the family members.

TROUBLESHOOTING TIPS FOR FAMILY ENGAGEMENT DIFFICULTIES

Objective

The purpose of this section is to help therapists anticipate common challenges to obtaining caregiver engagement and participation in the CM treatment process and to suggest strategies to address these difficulties.

Challenges and Solutions

First, it might be helpful to remember that, with few exceptions, challenges to the implementation of CM with substance-abusing youths and their families are generally the same as the challenges that arise in the treatment of other behavioral and emotional problems in adolescents. That is, barriers to implementation can include such factors as parental disagreement about how to handle a youth's discipline, caregiver depression, long work hours that interfere with monitoring capacity, lack of indigenous resources (e.g., social support, instrumental aid), caregiver substance abuse, and so forth. That said, a few implementation challenges are relatively common in families of substance-abusing adolescents. These challenges are identified next, as are strategies therapists might use to address them.

Caregivers Feel Put Off by the Amount of Time and Attention Needed to Conduct CM with the Youth.

The therapist might request that caregivers try the intervention for two or three sessions. The therapist and caregiver can learn from this participation if there are ways to make caregiver involvement in CM more efficient. The therapist can suggest that, as with all new skills, once the youth and caregiver have practiced a bit, the process will go more quickly. The therapist can also help caregivers establish a specific time of day they could work with the CM tasks, much as they would establish a specific time of day to help the youth with homework. In this way, the sense that a chore is hanging over their heads all day long can be diminished.

Another strategy is for therapists to find out from caregivers how much time they are currently spending dealing with the consequences of the youth's drug use. This might include time spent interfacing with agencies (i.e., schools, juvenile justice), following up on irresponsible behavior, monitoring, and generally doing things that would not be required if the adolescent was behaving responsibly. When caregivers realize how much time they already devote to dealing with the youth's drug use, they may be more willing to temporarily invest effort with the potential payoff of less work in the future.

Caregivers Contend That "It's Not My Problem" and That the Youth Should Be Solely Responsible for Completing Treatment.

Here the therapist might emphasize that although the caregivers were not the "cause" of the problem, they are most likely the youth's best hope for a favorable solution. The caregivers possess a degree of wisdom, maturity, and experience that can be critically important to helping the youth achieve abstinence. Although the caregivers might have good reasons for not wanting to be involved now, giving up all responsibility is simply not realistic (i.e., they will remain involved and important sources of competence building throughout their children's adolescence and adulthood) or good for the youth. Rather, utilization of the caregivers' skills and resources is essential to increasing the odds of success.

Caregivers Believe That Drug Use Is a Medical Condition That Should Be Treated Medically.

In this scenario, debating the extent to which drug use is a medical versus a behavioral condition is rarely helpful. The therapist can certainly agree that substance use makes changes in the brain and body without weighing in on the issue of whether drug use is a bona fide medical problem. The therapist can emphasize the following, however:

- The damaging effects of drug use and abuse on the health of the youth is another reason (i.e., in addition to the psychosocial problems experienced by the youth) to urgently try to stop drug use.
- Chronic medical conditions such as high blood pressure and diabetes need to be managed with changes in behavior, even when medications are used to help treat the condition. For example, people with diabetes often have to closely monitor the amount and types of foods they eat, make finger pricks throughout the day to check their blood sugar levels, and so forth. When the person with the illness is a child, the caregivers are largely responsible for ensuring that the child eats the right foods, checks his or her blood sugar level, takes medications on time, and so forth. That is, the caregivers help the child perform the tasks required to manage the illness so that problems don't get worse.

Caregivers Are Overwhelmed by Treatment Demands.

When caregivers feel overwhelmed with the complexity of treatment, the therapist might want to first find out more about their concerns, what stressors they are experiencing, and how they see these stressors as impacting their ability to participate in CM interventions. Often the initial process of starting CM can feel overwhelming as parents try to grasp the different components of treatment and adjust to a more active therapeutic role. One way to help caregivers is to break down the components of each task into smaller, more manageable steps and to reassure them that the therapist will be there to support them and provide assistance with each step of the intervention. For example, the therapist might agree to call the caregiver to remind him or her to do a step in treatment, walk the caregiver through a step over the phone, or model the step during a session. The central therapeutic goal in this process is to shape the caregivers' behavior by giving them small tasks in which they can be successful in their child's treatment and then gradually adding more assignments as their confidence increases.

Caregivers Have Limited Social Supports.

Some caregivers are overwhelmed with the demands on their time in caring for their family. For example, a single parent working 50 hours a week and raising several children might realistically have limited time for engaging in treatment with her 16-year-old son. Such caregivers (and their children) might benefit from increased social supports. Here the therapist might help the family identify potential resources within their own family and community whenever possible. Some basic steps for helping families build their social support resources, based on *The Ecology of Troubled Children* by Richard Munger (1998), are listed next.

Steps in Building Social Supports

- Help align the caregiver's goals with the need for social supports.
- Outline what some of the social support needs are now, especially as they apply to CM treatment.
- Help the caregiver identify all potential sources of support by brainstorming, without excluding any possible supports at first.
- Find out what the caregiver has already done to access social supports as well as barriers encountered.
- Match the family's list of specific needs with the list of potential sources of support. For example, uncle or grandmother might be able to drive youth and mom to appointments.
- Assess the pros and cons of each potential person in that role. For example, it makes the most sense to ask grandmother to drive as uncle works and is not as able to help.
- Decide how to address barriers to using that support. For example, grandmother is busy on all days but Friday, so the appointment will need to take place on Fridays.
- Determine the "cost" of accessing the support and develop a plan for reciprocating. For example, grandmother might start to feel that she is being taken for granted. She is tired on Fridays and might not want to keep driving to all the appointments. To address this possible limitation, the youth will wash grandmother's car twice a month, and the youth and caregiver will both thank grandmother and make dinner for her on Fridays after the appointment.
- Develop a concrete plan for how the family will approach the support person.
- Follow up with the family to monitor how the plan is being implemented.

Caregivers Feel the Youth Is Too Old to Need Such Intensive Parenting ("He/She Is Old Enough to Know Better").

The therapist will want to find out more about why the caregiver holds this belief. One or more of the following sets of information might be useful for the therapist depending on the caregiver's underlying beliefs.

Developmental Immaturity. While teens are often physically mature and might be very adult-like in their appearance, their brains are still immature and in the process of developing. In particular, the aspects of the human brain (frontal lobes) that govern judgment, insight, and rational decision making are some of the last areas to finish growing and are not fully developed until much later in life. Also, rational decision-making skills develop through practice and experience. As a result, youth who have a poor track record for making good decisions cannot be expected to develop these skills without guidance and practice.

Vulnerable Youth. Adolescents are often under a lot of pressure to use drugs. Staying off drugs requires good judgment, strong willpower, and social skills to avoid them. Just as some children learn to walk, talk, or read more slowly than others, many do not develop good judgment and decision-making skills until they are adults. As a result, some youth are more vulnerable to drug use than others, especially if they have been using drugs that, by their nature, slow the development of strong decision-making skills.

Parents Proven to Be the Best Intervention. Research has shown that adolescent drug use happens most often when teens have friends who use drugs. In turn, adolescents are most likely to hang out with drug-using friends when they do not have close supervision at home and when they have problems in school. This is good news because it means that caregivers have the power to change teen drug use. Research shows that when caregivers are able to monitor adolescents and keep them busy in school or other prosocial activities, their drug use goes down. The CM treatment process helps parents intervene with school, friends, or whatever is going on to drive drug use in their child.

A High Level of Negative Emotions between the Youth and Caregiver Interferes with the Implementation of CM.

Because substance abuse in youth is often accompanied by other criminal activities, school problems, and oppositional behaviors, a certain amount of negative affect between the adolescent and caregiver is to be expected. A small percentage of families, however, have excessively high levels of negative affect and cognitions as a result of their long history of coercive interactions. For these families, the therapist should consider how each intervention can be conducted despite the negative emotions. Thus, it might make the most sense for the therapist to meet with the caregiver and youth (either individually or together) to get a better understanding of what is driving the negative affect. When this issue is better understood, the therapist should establish an agreement, if possible, from both caregiver and youth to keep negative comments and behaviors to a minimum during sessions. Ideally, the sessions can be thought of as steps taken toward repairing the youth–caregiver relationship. For example, for caregivers who no longer trust their youth because of repeated lies and bad behaviors, CM can be a process that allows youth to regain trust through clean screens and work toward sobriety. Also, as caregivers start to better understand the youth's drug use, what drives that use, and what they can do to diminish that use, they may begin to feel more empowered. Youth might also benefit by participating in a treatment in which their caregivers reward them for clean screens. If negative emotions between the youth and caregiver continue to interfere with treatment, despite therapist intervention, the therapist should consider meeting with the youth and caregiver separately at first and then bringing them together to facilitate the sharing of information. In these instances, the therapist should strive to make sure that both parties have access to all information shared in treatment because a core aspect of CM involves empowering the caregivers to better understand what drives their child's drug use so that they can facilitate abstinence. Finally, high levels of negative family affect are frequently treated effectively by evidence-based family therapies. Although the present CM approach is family based, it is not a comprehensive family therapy. Thus, for families with persisting high levels of negative affect, the therapist should collaborate with or refer the family to a practitioner with evidence-based family therapy skills.

Caregivers Abuse Drugs or Have Serious Mental Health Problems.

Because adverse family and social contexts often play a substantial role in reinforcing youth drug use, the therapist might learn that the youth's caregiver is experiencing substance abuse or serious mental health problems. Some recommendations to help the therapist think through this challenge are listed next.

Caregivers Have Substance Abuse or Serious Mental Health Problems

- Share your knowledge or concern about the substance use/mental health problem with the caregiver in a manner that is supportive. Be careful to do this in a way that helps the caregiver maintain his or her parenting role.
- Meet individually with the caregiver to find out how his or her substance use/mental health problem impacts the youth's treatment.
- Align with the caregiver in working together to help the youth get clean, and try to anticipate how the caregiver's substance use/mental health concern might be a barrier for the youth. For example, if smelling marijuana is a trigger for the youth, then mom might trigger the youth to use drugs if she smokes marijuana in the house. Similarly, if mom sleeps in the afternoon rather than at night because of depression, how is she going to monitor her son after school?
- Work with the caregiver to find out what he or she is able to do if his or her substance use/mental health problem is a barrier or trigger for the youth.
- Develop a plan with the caregiver concerning how he or she would like to handle the youth's reference to the caregiver's drug use/mental health problem during sessions.
- Offer to assist the caregiver in obtaining treatment for his or her drug use/mental health problem as indicated.
- Overall, the goal is to support the caregiver in his or her role as a parent and to help the caregiver develop and maintain the authority to enforce rules and reward clean behaviors, while at the same time developing a process by which the youth can honestly share information during sessions concerning the caregiver's drug use/mental health problem.

THERAPIST CHECKLISTS FOR CHAPTER 3: INTRODUCING CONTINGENCY MANAGEMENT AND ENGAGING FAMILIES IN TREATMENT

THERAPIST CHECKLIST 3.1

Introducing Contingency Management

Case number: ______________ **Session date:** ______________

I have explained that (check each item covered in session):

___ CM is a type of treatment that has been proven to help people stop using drugs.

___ CM has been shown to help people who have alcohol or drug (marijuana, cocaine, and opium/heroin) dependence even when those problems have been long lasting.

___ This type of treatment will require work by both the youth in treatment and his/her caregiver(s).

___ The treatment has four parts, which I will help you to learn.

___ In the first part, we will learn about the people, places, feelings, and thoughts that influence or "trigger" [youth's name] drug/alcohol use.

___ Next, we will develop a list of activities and things [youth's name] would like to earn that will help motivate him/her to stay away from drugs/alcohol.

___ Once we have developed this list, we will sign a contract that will be like a working agreement between (*youth's name*) and us. In this contract, we will outline in detail what privileges and activities (*youth's name*) can earn in return for having clean drug screens and breath scans.

___ Urine drug screens and breath scans will need to be collected at least once a week at first to help us track how treatment is going. When the screens are clean, (*youth's name*) will earn points and rewards that are outlined in the contract.

___ Finally, we will help (*youth's name*) learn how to avoid drugs and deal with situations in which drug use is likely.

___ It will take us several sessions to learn these parts, but when you have learned them, you will both have the tools needed to reach your goals.

___ This program will take about 14 to 18 weeks to complete, depending on how many sessions we have each week and how (*youth's name*) progresses in treatment.

THERAPIST CHECKLIST 3.2

Engaging the Family in Treatment

Case number: ____________ **Session date:** ____________

This checklist is intended as a self-monitoring instrument to support therapist use of strategies that promote family collaboration in treatment. These strategies are *central to all treatment sessions* throughout the course of CM.

I have (check each strategy implemented or confirmed in session):

___ Engendered hope for treatment success among family members.

___ Collaborated with the family in the analysis of problems and design of interventions, rather than solely directing the analysis and design myself.

___ Made sure or confirmed that we (family members and myself) are all working toward the same goals.

___ Made sure that the treatment plans are clearly linked to the goals of the family.

___ Made sure that the family members understand how the planned CM interventions are specifically linked with their treatment goals.

___ Maintained a firm (an aim of treatment is to eliminate or reduce drug use) but positive (we can be successful if all work hard on this) stance.

___ Maintained a strength-focused approach with the youth and family, emphasizing the positive features of their functioning and therapeutic efforts.

Sample Dialogue: Introducing Contingency Management and Engaging Families in Treatment

TASKS 3.1 (INTRODUCING CONTINGENCY MANAGEMENT) AND 3.2 (ENGAGING THE FAMILY IN TREATMENT)

Therapist: Welcome, Tony, Ms. Smith. I see that you have brought someone with you.

Caregiver: Yes. This is my husband, Al.

Therapist: Nice to meet you, Mr. Smith.

Stepfather: You can call me Al.

Therapist: [addressing Tony] It looks as if you brought your whole family with you here today.

Tony: Yeah, now they can both get on my case.

Therapist: Hmmm . . .

Stepfather: [addressing Tony] Watch your mouth. I've taught you better than that.

Therapist: I can see that Tony seems a little unsure about you attending our session today, Mr. Smith, yet I want to tell you that I am personally very glad that you've come.

Tony: Yeah, now it's three against one.

Therapist: Tony, when you left last week, it felt to me like the three of us were starting to get to know each other and had started to develop a plan for working together to help you with your drug use. What happened?

Tony: What do you think? He [pointing at stepfather] happened.

Caregiver: Let me see if I can explain. Last week when I got home, I started telling Al about what we were doing in treatment and I guess I got confused. Al started asking a lot of questions that I couldn't answer, and so finally I decided to take you up on your offer and bring him with us. Thanks for rescheduling on short notice.

Therapist: No problem. This is actually a perfect session for Al to attend because I'm going to be explaining everything about the treatment to you today.

Tony: [addressing his mother] You didn't tell her what Al said.

Stepfather: I'll tell you what I said. I told my wife that this didn't sound like any sort of treatment I had heard of before. You've already met with them twice, and I know Tony is still using.

Tony: Am not.

Stepfather: You must think I'm stupid. You might pull things over on your mother, but I know what you are up to. I saw how red your eyes were last Friday night.

Therapist: Al, it's good to see how concerned you are about Tony's well-being. I learned from your wife last week that you have been helping with Tony since he was young, about 6 I think?

Stepfather: Yeah, he was 6 when we married. I've always tried to treat him like my own son. I guess he is my only son. I've got a grown daughter, but he's my only boy.

Therapist: Good, I'm glad you are around because Tony and his mother are going to need help as we try to accomplish our mutual goal of helping Tony get off drugs and alcohol.

Stepfather: So, how exactly are you planning to do this?

Therapist: Well, actually it helps if you think of it as all of us working together to help Tony.

Stepfather: Seems to me that it should be his responsibility [pointing at Tony, Tony rolling his eyes in response] since he is the one using.

Therapist: Yes, at some level that would seem to make sense. Yet this program that I am going to talk about today, contingency management or CM, takes a slightly different approach.

Stepfather: What do you mean?

Therapist: In CM, we work with families to help youth get off drugs. We have found that teenagers respond best to treatment when family members play an active role in helping the youth get off drugs.

Stepfather: How are we supposed to help?

Therapist: Good question. You are actually helping now.

Tony: [Mumbles.] You call this help?

Therapist: Yes. Attending sessions is the first step, just like your family is doing now. As caregivers participate in treatment, they start to understand what things are going on in their teen's life that may be triggering him to try and use drugs and so they can help their child strategize and develop plans for dealing with drug use. Parents help their youth by rewarding him when he is clean.

Stepfather: What about punishment?

Therapist: Yes, you withhold rewards when your son uses and reward him when he is clean.

Stepfather: The old carrot and stick.

Therapist: Yes, and we've found that emphasizing the rewards, or carrots, is a good approach to take with teenagers.

Caregiver: Is that because teens are so rebellious and hate it when you punish them?

Therapist: Yes, that's exactly right. Teens are at a unique place in their development. While they may look and act like adults in many ways, they are still growing and learning. That is one of the reasons that they still need parents to be very actively involved in many aspects of their lives, including treatment.

Stepfather: What about the stick? Spare the rod, spoil the child, as my old man used to say.

Therapist: That's also a good point. I didn't mean to imply that we would coddle Tony or shower him with rewards for no reason. This treatment hinges on parents creating a lot of structure for their teen. By structure, I mean that the parents help set up rules for how the youth will be rewarded when he is clean, and they must stick to those rules. So, for instance, if Tony has to have clean drug screens to use his cell phone and he tests dirty that week, it's the parents' job to make sure he doesn't have his cell phone until he tests clean again.

Stepfather: So how does this all work?

Therapist: [Follows *Therapist Checklist 3.1: Introducing Contingency Management.*] Okay, let me start from the beginning. Contingency management, or CM, is the type of treatment we will be providing for Tony. A lot of research has been done on CM, and it has been shown to help people get off drugs and alcohol.

Stepfather: Sort of like AA?

Therapist: Actually more than AA. There is substantially more research to support CM, especially with youth, than to support AA.

Stepfather: I think AA works. It worked for my father.

Therapist: Yes, some people find AA to be very helpful, yet the approach we will use here is somewhat different.

Caregiver: Al, would you please stop interrupting?

Therapist: No, please, questions are important. Do you have any, Ms. Smith?

Caregiver: No, Al has asked all the ones I can think of, and then some.

Therapist: Let me tell you some more about CM. There are basically four parts to CM, and I will teach you each of these parts. Once we have learned each part, we will put them all together each week in every session.

Tony: You mean like four lessons?

Therapist: That's a good comparison. In the first lesson or part of CM, we'll spend some time trying to understand what things in Tony's life might be triggering him to want to use drugs.

Tony: Things?

Therapist: By things, I mean what sorts of people, places, situations, and feelings might happen just before you use drugs. When they look at it closely, most people find that there are events that frequently occur right before they use, events that lead them to use.

Stepfather: Are you trying to say that outside forces are causing Tony to use? How about his inside force, his desire to get high, avoid work, escape the hard facts of life?

Therapist: Well, yes, as you just stated, there may be things he is trying to avoid or escape, things that are hard or unpleasant. Those can all be triggers.

Caregiver: Al, you should know all about that. You smoke cigarettes.

Therapist: Let's take cigarette smoking as an example. Mr. Smith, would that be okay?

Stepfather: Sure, go for it.

Therapist: Can you think of things that happen to you during the day that increase your chances of smoking?

Caregiver: Like getting out of bed in the morning, right after you drink your coffee.

Stepfather: I guess. I usually smoke right after my morning coffee.

Tony: You smoke after supper too, and whenever you and mom fight, you always go out on the porch and smoke one.

Stepfather: I have to smoke two when I fight with you.

Therapist: You guys are right on target. This is exactly what I am talking about. So, in the first lesson, we will be working with Tony to try and figure out what kinds of things may trigger him to use drugs or alcohol.

Tony: What comes next?

Therapist: The second lesson involves helping Tony create plans for dealing with his triggers. So, continuing with the cigarette example, we might plan with you, Mr. Smith, to take a walk or do something else with that stress you feel after fighting.

Stepfather: How about take away the source, fighting.

Therapist: Yes, that too. We might help your family come up with ways to fight less so you would be less likely to use.

Tony: What do we call that lesson?

Therapist: Self-management planning. Then, in the next session, or lesson, your family will sign a contract. The contract will outline Tony's roles and responsibilities in CM and how he can earn rewards and privileges when he is able to be clean from drug use.

Stepfather: So we will reward Tony when he is clean? How will we reward him?

Therapist: Part of this lesson is figuring out how to reward Tony. To do this, we will sit down with Tony and find out what sorts of things he currently gets from you guys and . . .

Stepfather: Like his cell phone?

Therapist: Right. We will figure out what things you already give him and what sorts of additional things he may be willing to work for.

Stepfather: Sounds expensive. Am I supposed to finance this?

Therapist: Well, yes and no. This is the most common concern that families have, and so I want to reassure you that we will all work together to make sure that the rewards are affordable yet meaningful. It is important that they be something Tony is motivated to earn.

Stepfather: He has expensive taste. I'm a little worried about that.

Therapist: Yes, most teens do, and I promise that you and your wife will have final say about the items that are put on the list. Many families realize, when participating in this lesson, that they already give their youth many things, so some of this lesson is learning to tie those "gifts" or rewards to good behavior.

Tony: Hey, sounds like I am getting tricked.

Therapist: Don't worry. We will do our best to make sure you get rewarded when you work hard.

Caregiver: Is it sort of like paying Tony for work?

Therapist: Yes, that is exactly right. In this treatment model, we often like to think of getting off drugs as hard work.

Caregiver: I know about that. I stopped smoking cigarettes about 5 years ago, and it was about the hardest thing I've ever done. Maybe we can try this on you Al, with your cigarettes.

Stepfather: If Tony will stop using that will probably reduce my stress to about half, so I will probably smoke less. By the way, how are we going to know if Tony is using?

Therapist: That brings us to the fourth lesson: drug screens.

Caregiver: Right. I am sort of worried about this one.

Therapist: We will be screening Tony for drug and alcohol use periodically throughout the treatment.

Stepfather: What do you mean by screening?

Therapist: In the fourth lesson, I will be teaching you how to collect urine drug screens and alcohol breath scans on Tony. Each week, or potentially several times a week, one of us will collect these. If they are clean, Tony will earn points and privileges. If they are dirty, he will lose privileges and fail to gain points.

Caregiver: So we have to collect those, at our house?

Therapist: Ideally yes, as the best time to collect screens is right after high-risk situations. So, for instance, if Al thinks Tony's eyes are red when he comes in on Saturday night, he could have Tony provide a urine screen and breath scan for us. If Tony is clean, he gets points. If he's dirty, he loses privileges.

Stepfather: What if he refuses?

Therapist: Then we assume the results are dirty.

Caregiver: Is the screen hard to do?

Therapist: The cups are designed to be easy to use. I'll be able to show you, and you will have a handout describing what to do. Also, you can always call me if you run into trouble.

Stepfather: Okay, that's four lessons. Then what?

Therapist: So, after you have learned the four lessons or components, then we will do each one every time we meet.

Tony: What do you mean? Does that mean the sessions will take forever?

Therapist: So, you will come in and I will find out the results of the last drug screen. If the results are dirty, then we will try and find out what sorts of things may have triggered or led to the use. Next, we will make sure that the rewards and consequences are being carried out correctly. Finally, we will help you think through ways to modify your self-management plans based on the triggers and what went wrong the prior week. If you need help with anything, like skills for telling your friends you don't want to use, we will work on those things.

Tony: What if the screens are clean?

Therapist: Then usually the sessions are somewhat easier, yet we still look at the last week, what triggers occurred, how you and your family managed them, and then we modify the self-management plans if we think they need it. We may still work on things like skills too. Of course, the best part is that I make sure the rewards work for you and that you can buy things with your points if you like.

Caregiver: Sounds very practical. I could have used something like this when I was trying to quit smoking.

Stepfather: Okay, sounds good, I'm sold. How long will this take?

Therapist: This treatment takes about 14 to 18 weeks from this point forward. The amount of time it takes depends on a lot of different things, including how often we meet, how much work we get done in each session, and Tony's response to treatment. So, for example, if Tony gets clean quickly and stays clean, then we may be done 3 months from now. If, on the other hand, it takes us longer to help him get clean and sustain sobriety, we can go much longer. There is no limit here at the clinic for how long we can go.

Caregiver: How long do most kids take?

Therapist: It varies greatly, yet many can be done with 14 to 18 weeks of hard work.

Therapist: Let me ask one thing. I meant to do this earlier and forgot. Ms. Smith, Tony, and I talked about our goals for treatment last week. Can you tell me what you would like for Tony to accomplish in therapy?

Stepfather: I want him to get off drugs, stay in school, and stop stressing me and his mother out.

Therapist: Sounds like the same goals we came up with last week. Do you agree, Ms. Smith?

Caregiver: Yes, Al and I are on the same page about this.

Therapist: Tony, I think you had similar goals. Do you remember them?

Tony: I want to get off probation, not go to prison.

Therapist: Something else? Something involving work, sports?

Tony: Oh yeah, I hope that by getting clean, I can do better at basketball and stay in school easier.

Therapist: That way you will be more likely to graduate from school.

Caregiver: He will also be more likely to get a job. I want Tony to grow into the responsible adult I know is in him.

Therapist: Well said. Let's end on that note today.

CHAPTER 4

ABC Assessment of Drug Use

THERAPIST GOALS

1. **Introduce the ABC assessment and explain how to identify triggers for substance use.**
2. **Complete the ABC assessment with the youth and caregiver.**

The therapist teaches the youth and caregiver to conduct an ABC assessment of the youth's drug use. An ABC assessment is used to identify events in the environment that occur before, during, and after drug use. In conducting this assessment, the therapist, youth, and caregiver focus on three phases of behavior: the ABCs:

1. **A**ntecedents (i.e., triggers or cues for drug use).
2. **B**ehavior (i.e., actions leading to use, drug use itself).
3. **C**onsequences (i.e., reinforcement, punishment) of the behavior.

OVERVIEW OF THE ABC ASSESSMENT

The basic rationale of the ABC assessment (Budney & Higgins, 1998) is that drug use is triggered by certain events, situations, and feelings and maintained by immediate and long-term consequences. An ABC assessment of drug use, therefore, identifies:

1. Triggers, which can be people, places, and activities that are present consistently before or during drug use.
2. Thoughts and feelings that prompt or lead to drug use.
3. Drug use behavior.
4. Short- and long-term consequences, both positive and negative, that influence drug use.

Each of these concepts is described in more detail next.

Identification of Triggers for Drug Use

Triggers or antecedents (the *A* in *ABC*) are things that occur right before a youth uses drugs or that lead to drug use cravings. Almost anything can be a trigger. Some triggers are easy to identify, and others are harder to figure out. Triggers can be particular people, places, feelings, situations, or a mixture of these that can make someone want to use drugs. For example, triggers might include seeing an empty warehouse where youth get together to smoke marijuana, smelling marijuana on the jacket of a friend, or hearing others talk about a party where drugs will be used.

Thoughts and Feelings Related to Drug Use

Drug use triggers can lead to thoughts and feelings about using drugs, and these can further evoke drug use. Examples of some thoughts that might trigger drug use are "I am going to feel so good. I can't wait to get high because I am going to have so much fun"; "I need to forget about her or him" (after breaking up with a boyfriend or girlfriend); and "I can't deal with all this nagging. Let me get out of here to get high." Feelings that trigger drug use might include boredom, anxiety about an upcoming test or going out on a date, nervousness about meeting someone, fear, loneliness, or happiness.

Drug Use Itself

Drug use is one of the many behaviors that a youth might demonstrate after experiencing a trigger. Drug use behaviors (the *B* in *ABC*) can include drug seeking ("I went to Dan's house to get a bag of weed") and use ("When I was at Dan's house I smoked a blunt"). It is important to help the youth list all his or her drug-using behaviors, including their frequency and duration. For example, drug use behaviors that would be listed in the *B* category of the ABC assessment might include obtaining money to buy drugs, contacting a drug supplier, and plotting when and where to use the drugs once obtained. This aspect of the assessment should also include behaviors designed to avoid detection of use, such as burning incense, using cologne, and chewing gum.

Consequences of Drug Use

Extensive research on human behavior has shown that what happens as a result of a behavior, its consequences (the *C* in *ABC*), affects the odds that an individual will engage in the behavior again. A consequence that increases the odds a behavior will occur again is called a *reinforcer*. For example, feeling good, enjoying the company of friends, and experiencing relief from physical or psychological pain are some consequences of drug use that typically increase the odds an individual will use drugs again. These are, therefore, reinforcers of drug use.

A consequence that decreases the odds a behavior will occur again is called a *punisher.* A punisher can be an aversive consequence for a behavior, such as having to do extra chores or getting arrested. The removal of reinforcement for a behavior, such as loss of privileges or an allowance, also can have a punishing effect (i.e., decrease the odds of the behavior occurring again). Thus, there are two kinds of punishers: (1) the presence of an aversive consequence and (2) the removal of a reinforcer. Negative consequences associated with adolescent drug use can include such outcomes as getting arrested, getting kicked out of school, poor grades, arguments or fights with parents, arguments or fights with friends, disappointing one's parents, losing the opportunity to play a sport, losing a job, and failing a test. Unfortunately, most negative consequences occur so far after the drug use event that they have little or no influence on immediate drug consumption.

Aims and Time Frame of the Following Tasks

The primary goal of the following tasks is to help the youth and caregiver become more familiar with the concept of triggers and to begin to identify the events or antecedents that might either increase or decrease the youth's chances of using drugs or alcohol. In addition, the youth and caregiver will learn how to identify the positive and negative consequences of instances of substance use. Ideally, the therapist will be able to complete this set of tasks in a single 1-hour session and give the family a homework assignment of completing a blank *ABC Assessment* worksheet (Form 4.2) on one other instance of drug use before the next session.

THERAPIST TASK 4.1: INTRODUCING THE ABC ASSESSMENT AND EXPLAINING HOW TO IDENTIFY TRIGGERS OF SUBSTANCE USE

Objectives

1. Explain that a clear picture of what maintains the youth's drug use is needed before the youth can be helped to stop using drugs.
2. Introduce the ABC assessment as a useful tool for getting that clear picture.
3. Introduce the features of the ABC assessment.
4. Teach the youth and caregiver to identify triggers for recent drug use with *Discovering Triggers of Your Substance Use* (Form 4.1).

Materials

- *Therapist Checklist 4.1: Introducing the ABC Assessment*
- *Discovering Triggers of Your Substance Use* (Form 4.1)

Accomplishing the Objectives

Following the steps outlined in *Therapist Checklist 4.1: Introducing the ABC Assessment*, the therapist starts by sitting down with the youth and caregiver, introducing the concept of the ABC assessment, and providing a *Discovering Triggers of Your Substance Use* worksheet (Form 4.1). The youth is encouraged to complete the form, and the therapist and caregiver go over it with the youth. Some flexibility about whether the form is filled out by the youth or completed by the therapist using an interview style is allowed. The clinical goals are to (1) help the caregiver and youth *both* start to obtain a better understanding of the concept of "triggers" and how events in the environment can either increase or decrease the likelihood that drug use will occur and (2) get the caregiver and youth engaged in treatment and communicating about the youth's drug use in solution-focused ways. Once *Discovering Triggers of Your Substance Use* (Form 4.1) is completed, the therapist moves to Therapist Task 4.2, which is to complete an *ABC Assessment* (Form 4.2) with the family.

THERAPIST TASK 4.2: COMPLETING THE ABC ASSESSMENT

Objective

1. Teach the youth to identify the triggers, thoughts, feelings, and consequences for a recent drug use incident.

Materials

- *Therapist Checklist 4.2: Completing the ABC Assessment*
- *ABC Assessment* (Form 4.2)
- *The ABCs of Drug Use* (Handout 4.1)

Accomplishing the Objective

After *Discovering Triggers of Your Substance Use* (Form 4.1) is completed (Therapist Task 4.1), the therapist shifts into the second task, which is to complete an *ABC Assessment* (Form 4.2) with the family. The primary aim of this exercise is for the youth and caregiver to better understand how antecedents or triggers lead to substance-using behaviors and that these, in turn, have positive and negative consequences for the youth and family. To accomplish this aim, the therapist follows the steps outlined in *Therapist Checklist 4.2: Completing the ABC Assessment*. A blank *ABC Assessment* (Form 4.2) and an example worksheet (*The ABCs of Drug Use* [Handout 4.1]) are provided to both the youth and caregiver. The therapist then asks the youth to think about the last time he or she used a drug and to help the therapist fill out the form. The appropriate antecedents or triggers identified previously on *Discovering Triggers of Your Substance Use* (Form 4.1) can be listed in column "A." Then the therapist works with the family to complete columns

"B" and "C." The items listed in column "B" are details of both drug use behaviors (e.g., rolling a blunt) and those behaviors that lead to drug use (e.g., obtaining money, calling a friend to plan use). Items in column "C" are the short- and long-term consequences that increase or decrease the chances of substance use in the future. It is often helpful to go over *The ABCs of Drug Use* (Handout 4.1) with the participants. When the objectives of this task are accomplished, the therapist should probably give the family a homework assignment of completing a blank *ABC Assessment* (Form 4.2) on one other instance of drug use before the next session. After all components of CM have been introduced, the family and therapist will complete an *ABC Assessment* (Form 4.2) on a routine basis during each session to understand the youth's drug use or abstinence based on the results of random drug tests.

TROUBLESHOOTING TIPS

Objective

The purpose of this section is to help therapists anticipate common challenges to conducting the ABC assessment and to suggest strategies to address these difficulties.

Challenges and Solutions

The Youth Has Difficulty Identifying Drug Use Triggers.

The therapist can acknowledge that, for someone who has used drugs for a while, it can be a little tricky at first to identify triggers of use. The therapist might frame the task as a kind of detective work to be done together until the youth and caregiver get more practice doing it on their own. The therapist can then introduce several tools for helping with the detective work.

- First, ask the youth to recall the last time he or she used drugs and use that instance as a reference point for completing each of the worksheets.
- Second, ask the youth to self-monitor future instances of drug use and record triggers, behaviors, and consequences associated with each instance.
- Third, the therapist might need to suggest, on the basis of his or her assessment of the youth's ecology (i.e., family, peer, school, neighborhood, and community context), possible antecedents of use.
- Fourth, the therapist might need to suggest antecedents for substance use that have been identified by other adolescents and examine similarities between these antecedents and any aspect of the people, places, activities, thoughts, or feelings the youth experienced just before using drugs or while using them. The similarities might not be immediately obvious to the youth. The therapist might need to volunteer best guesses about aspects of the environment surrounding the youth that seem similar to aspects of the environment identified by other adolescents as triggers for their drug use.

The Youth Is Reluctant to Share Information Concerning His or Her Drug Use.

When the youth does not want to admit or discuss current drug use, the therapist has at least three options.

- Ask the youth to describe drug use situations that occurred in the more distant past, and try to complete *Discovering Triggers of Your Substance Use* (Form 4.1) and the *ABC Assessment* (Form 4.2) for those situations.
- Ask the youth to think of a friend who uses drugs and try to think of triggers for the friend's drug use.
- Ask the youth to complete the ABC assessment procedures with little detail at first, and gradually get the youth to include greater detail in subsequent sessions as trust is established.

The Youth is Reluctant to Share Information about His or Her Peers.

Because affiliation with peers who use drugs is often a powerful driver of youth drug use, it is ultimately very important to understand the role of peers in supporting both drug use and abstinence for the youth. Often teens are reluctant to share this information early in treatment. Common reasons are presented next, along with some potential strategies for approaching the problem.

Don't Want to "Snitch." It is normal for adolescents to be very reluctant to give information to authority figures (i.e., therapist, caregiver) that might get their friends in trouble. As a result, therapists might reassure youth concerning the confidentiality of the information they provide during sessions.

Don't Want the Caregiver to Know. Similar to the first concern, youth might be worried that their caregivers will get their friends in trouble or restrict the youth's access to these friends. This fear is actually warranted, as a goal of treatment is to find out about drug-using peers and limit the adolescent's access to them. One way to address these concerns is to get agreement from the caregiver and youth together on acceptable caregiver responses to peer information. While the caregiver cannot promise to let the youth continue to be with these peers unsupervised, she or he might be able to agree not to call the parents of peers or to keep information confidential from other neighbors or friends.

Afraid the Caregiver Will Become Angry or Express Negative Affect. This is often a legitimate concern as caregivers frequently feel frustrated and powerless about their child's substance use behavior as they enter treatment. Therefore, the therapist might meet with the caregiver ahead of time to gain an understanding of possible frustrations and help coach him or her on how to reach the goals of early sessions (i.e., to get a good understanding of factors driving drug use). During this meeting, the therapist should engage the caregiver in a collaborative effort to provide a hopeful and supportive stance during sessions involving the youth. Some caregivers will benefit from practice and role plays to help model appropriate responses to in-session behaviors that are likely to be displayed by their child.

Continue to Refuse to Provide Specific Names Despite Interventions. Sometimes, despite good therapeutic effort, youth continue to refuse to give out details about the role of friends in their drug use. Such behavior should not be allowed to interfere with treatment. Rather, the therapist and caregiver might accept the youth's refusal for now, but let the youth know that they remain hopeful and predict that over time the youth will feel more comfortable sharing this information. One strategy for getting at least partial peer information from the youth includes allowing him or her to use code names or labels instead of real names to reference peers. For instance, the youth might call Joe "J" for the purposes of treatment. The idea behind this strategy is that if "J" is an important trigger, over time the therapist and caregiver will be able to find out enough information about "J" to develop interventions. Another strategy is to ask the youth to elaborate more on prosocial peers as outlined in the *Discovering Triggers of Your Substance Use* worksheet (Form 4.1). In this way, caregivers can at least begin to deduce which youth are safe and supportive of the teen's abstinence. Ultimately, as CM treatment progresses and the youth becomes motivated to gain rewards and is more trusting of the therapeutic process, he or she often becomes more willing to divulge important peer information.

Caregivers or Youth Have Difficulty Understanding CM Material.

The therapist should take into account the developmental status of the youth and caregivers. For youth and caregivers who struggle, are poorly educated, or have low intellectual functioning, therapists might want to simplify language, be more concrete, and avoid analogies. Sentences should express one main idea at a time. Use simple words and examples to explain the concepts. Often it works best to skip explanations and progress directly to the forms and worksheets.

THERAPIST CHECKLISTS, FORMS, AND HANDOUT FOR CHAPTER 4: ABC ASSESSMENT OF DRUG USE

THERAPIST CHECKLIST 4.1

Introducing the ABC Assessment

Case number: ______________ **Session Date:** ______________

I have explained that (check each item covered in session):

___ The ABC assessment is a tool that will help us better understand (*youth's name*) drug use, so that we can work together to help him/her stop using drugs.

___ The ABC assessment is broken into three parts that correspond with the letters *A, B*, and *C*.

___ **A = Antecedents**—or triggers—things that may make a person more likely to use drugs. These may be people, places, thoughts, feelings, and circumstances.

___ **B = Behavior**—what a person does to obtain or use drugs, such as getting money, going to meet the dealer, or smoking a blunt.

___ **C = Consequences**—what happens (good and bad) after a person uses drugs.

___ We will take what is learned from doing the ABC assessment and use the information to help [youth's name] make plans to stay clean.

___ (*Caregiver's name*), you and I will help (*youth's name*) learn to control what happens after a trigger so drug/alcohol use is less likely to occur the next time he/she experiences the trigger.

___ We will help (*youth's name*) make plans to avoid drug/alcohol-using friends and spend more time in healthy situations.

___ We will help (*youth's name*) learn an effective way to say "no" to people who offer him/her drugs/alcohol.

___ It is very possible that (*youth's name*) may slip up and use drugs/alcohol while trying to stop.

___ While we don't want (*youth's name*) to slip, we will consider slips as opportunities, and try to learn from them so they will be less likely to happen next time.

___ It will take some practice for us to get good at doing an ABC assessment together; most people find these helpful after they have tried one or two.

___ Now, let's get started with the first worksheet. [Hand out *Discovering Triggers of Your Substance Use* (Form 4.1).]

___ This form will help you better understand what things may serve as triggers for drug/alcohol use.

___ Let's go over the form together for a minute. [Go over with client and caregiver to ensure they understand and can read the form. Walk them through the material if they need assistance.]

(cont.)

___ Notice that the end of the form also pays attention to people, places, and situations that help your child not to use drugs. These questions are very important. We will use them to build a plan to help (*youth's name*) stay clean.

___ [Client completes form with assistance as needed.]

___ Now, let's go over the form. [Elicit information and assist the client so that a better understanding of the youth's triggers is obtained.]

___ [Consider having the family complete this form as a homework assignment if indicated.]

THERAPIST CHECKLIST 4.2

Completing the ABC Assessment

Case number: ______________ **Session Date:** ______________

I have explained that (check each item covered in session):

[Note: *Although this form primarily addresses the youth, caregiver participation should be encouraged and interwoven in the assessment process.*]

___ Now that we have a better sense of what triggers (*youth's name*)'s drug/alcohol use, we are going to complete the rest of the ABC assessment. Here is a form that will help as well as some information about how that form might be completed.

___ [Hand out *ABC Assessment* (Form 4.2) and *The ABCs of Drug Use* (Handout 4.1).]

___ First, I'll need for you (addressing youth) to think of the last time you used drugs/alcohol. This will help us fill out the form.

___ Tell me about the last time you used—and I will put that down here, in the "behavior column."

___ Okay, now let's look at what was going on right before you used. What sort of triggers did you experience? [Record in Antecedents (Triggers) column—use information obtained from *Discovering Triggers of Your Substance Use* (Form 4.1).]

___ Now, tell me about any thoughts or feelings that happened right after the triggers. [Record in Thoughts and Feelings section.]

___ Let's go over the behaviors again. Describe not only the drug/alcohol use but also anything you did to be able to use the drugs/alcohol. [Record in the Behaviors (Actions) column.]

___ Okay, next we need to think about what sort of consequences the drug/alcohol use had for you. Let's start with the good ones.

___ Tell me some positive things that happened after your drug/alcohol use. How did it help you?

___ Next, what were some bad things that happened because of your drug/alcohol use?

___ (*Caregiver's name*), let's make sure we get your input here [fill in caregiver information in the appropriate columns].

___ This is very helpful. We are going to use this information to help make plans to stop your drug use soon.

___ [Consider assigning homework to complete *ABC Assessment* (Form 4.2) for one more instance of substance use and for one of nonuse.]

FORM 4.1

Discovering Triggers of Your Substance Use

Client: ______________________________ Date: ______________

1. List the **places** where you are most likely to use substances (examples: ***during trips to the mall, on the corner, under the bleachers at the park, in the restroom at school***).

2. List the **people** with whom you are most likely to use substances (examples: ***friends who also use***).

3. List any **times** or **days** when you are more likely to use substances (examples: ***at night, during lunch time at school, or Friday nights, when my mother is at work***).

Example answers to the questions are in bold italic type. Adapted from Budney and Higgins (1998).

(cont.)

4. List any **activities or events** that make it more likely that you will use substances (examples: ***going to the store, arguing with parents, parties with friends***).

5. Do you think that you use substances when you are **feeling** certain ways or are in certain **situations**? Read through the following list and mark the ones that seem relevant to you. For those you have marked, list specific examples from your own experience.

   a. At the end of (or during) a tense day

   b. When faced with something you fear

   c. When you did poorly in school (e.g., failed a math test)

   d. When you have been taken advantage of

   e. When you are bored

   f. When you are in a social situation

   g. When you feel bad about yourself (e.g., "I'll never be good enough")

   h. When you are depressed or feel sad

   i. When you want to feel energized

   j. When you are faced with a tough decision (e.g., breaking up)

   k. When you want to be friendly

   l. When you wish your personality was different (e.g., more outgoing, cool)

   m. Others not listed here:

(cont.)

6. List the **places** where you are **unlikely** to use substances (examples: **at home, at school**).

7. List the **people** with whom you are **unlikely** to use substances (examples: **family members, members of church youth group, girlfriend/boyfriend**).

8. List the **times** or **days** when you are **unlikely** to use substances (examples: ***during the school day, when my mother is not working, on the weekend during the day***).

9. List the **activities** you are engaged in when you are **unlikely** to use substances (examples: ***spending time with family in specific activities, practicing with athletic team, going to school***).

FORM 4.2

ABC Assessment

Name: ______________________ **Date:** ____________

Drug of choice: ______________________________

Use this form to help figure out the triggers (antecedents), actions (behaviors), and good and bad outcomes (consequences) of the last time you used drugs. Fill out one of these forms for each of the drugs you use.

A		B		C
Antecedents (Triggers)	⇨	Behaviors (Actions)	⇨	Consequences (Outcomes): Good and Bad
Thoughts and Feelings:				

Adapted from Budney and Higgins (1998).

HANDOUT 4.1

The ABCs of Drug Use

The *A* (Antecedent): Triggers for drug use		**The *B* (Behavior):** Drug use itself	**The *C* (Consequences):** Positive or negative consequences of drug use
Things that occur right before a youth uses drugs or that lead to drug use cravings. These can be particular people, places, activities, feelings, thoughts, situations, or a mixture of these that make a youth want to use drugs. ***Thoughts and feelings*** can be a part of multiple triggers that further evoke drug use.		Includes drug *seeking* and drug *ingestion*. For drug *seeking*, list what youth did to obtain the drug. For drug *ingestion*, list what youth ingested and how much.	Things or experiences that happen after drug use. *Positive consequences* increase the likelihood of future drug use. *Negative consequences* decrease the likelihood of future drug use.
Examples of triggers: • Seeing an empty warehouse where peers get together to smoke pot • Smelling pot on the jacket of a friend • Hearing others talk about a party where drugs will be used	**Examples of *thoughts*** that might trigger use: "I am going to feel so good." "We are going to have a good time." "I need to forget about her/him." (after breaking up with a boyfriend or girlfriend) "I can't deal with all this nagging. Let me get out of here to get high." **Examples of *feelings*** that might trigger use: • Boredom • Fear • Anxiety about an upcoming test • Happiness • Nervousness about meeting someone • Loneliness	**Examples of drug seeking:** "Called John to find out if he had some pot." "Took some money from my sister's purse so I could buy drugs." **Examples of drug ingestion:** "Shared a blunt with Jimmy." "Took three to four drags off a joint when it was passed around—there were six of us sharing it."	**Examples of positive consequences (*reinforcers*):** • Feeling good • Enjoying the company of friends • Filling time with something fun/exciting • Experiencing relief from physical or psychological pain **Examples of negative consequences (*punishers*):** • Something bad gets added (i.e., extra chores) • Something good gets taken away (i.e., lose driving privileges)

The basic rationale of the ABC assessment is that drug use (the **B**ehavior of ABC) is triggered by certain events, situations, and feelings (the **A**ntecedents of ABC); and maintained by immediate and long-term consequences (the **C**onsequences of ABC).

Sample Dialogues: ABC Assessment

THERAPIST TASK 4.1: INTRODUCING ABC ASSESSMENT AND EXPLAINING HOW TO IDENTIFY TRIGGERS OF SUBSTANCE USE

Therapist: [to Tony and his mother, Ms. Smith] The treatment we will be doing together, contingency management, has four parts. The first part that we will learn in our session today is called the ABC assessment. The ideas behind ABC assessments are pretty straightforward. An ABC assessment is a way to figure out what things make Tony more likely to use drugs and what things make him less likely. One way to remember how to do an ABC assessment is to think of the ABCs:

- **The *A* stands for antecedent.** Antecedents are triggers or things that happen just before you use drugs. Triggers can be things you see or smell, such as pot on someone's coat. They can also be people, such as the person you get high with. Triggers can also be feelings such as sadness, or triggers can even be situations that make it more likely for you to use drugs, such as skipping class.
- **The *B* stands for behavior.** Behavior is what you do to get the drug as well as use the drug.

Therapist: Tony, can you think of some behavior that someone may do to get a drug?

Tony: Call a friend who smokes pot.

Therapist: Yep, that is a good example.

- **The *C* stands for consequences.** These are things that happen after you use drugs. Some consequences make you more likely to use, such as feeling high and having fun with your friends. However, some consequences may make you less likely to use, such as getting in trouble or being put on probation.

Tony: Yeah, my mom yells at me if she knows I've been smoking.

Caregiver: Plus you get everybody in the family upset, which is a big consequence for us. Tony and his stepfather really argue when my husband thinks Tony has been smoking.

Therapist: You guys are right on target. These are the kinds of things we will want to write down in Tony's ABC assessment in a minute.

Tony: So why do we have to do all of this?

Therapist: The idea behind all of this work is that once we understand what things trigger you to use drugs, then we can help you make plans, which are called self-management plans, to deal with those triggers.

Tony: I don't know about this trigger stuff. I use drugs when I decide to use. It don't have anything to do with triggers. Triggers are for guns.

Therapist: How do you get a gun to work?

Tony: Pull its trigger.

Therapist: Exactly. I'm trying to say that there may be things happening in your environment that make you want to use. Things that happen right before you decide that you feel like using. In other words, without you thinking about it, there may be things that trigger your brain to tell you to use.

Tony: I don't know. Seems pretty weird.

Caregiver: Tony, please be respectful.

Therapist: It's okay. I want Tony to ask questions since he is going to have to work hard to get off of drugs. I want to make sure he understands what he's supposed to do. Tony, I've got a worksheet here that I would like to go over with you and your mom. I think it may help to answer some questions you seem to have about triggers.

Tony: Okay.

Therapist: [Hands Tony and his mother each a copy of *Discovering Triggers of Your Substance Use* (Form 4.1).] I'd like you to look at this form, *Discovering Triggers of Your Substance Use* [Form 4.1], and write down at least two triggers for each of the first three items. As I said earlier, triggers are things that happen, or things that are around when Tony decides to use drugs. They can be people, places, and activities. Ms. Smith, it helps if parents look at the form and try to guess what their child might write down. Sometimes parents have a better idea of their child's drug use triggers than they realize. Of course, we are also hoping to find out about triggers that you or even Tony may not have known about before. [Tony and his mother both complete the first three items on the form.]

Tony: Here you go.

Therapist: Okay, looking at the form, for the first one, you put John's house. Tell me how being at John's house is a trigger.

Tony: John smokes pot and he usually asks me to smoke too.

Therapist: Tell me a little more about that. Are his parents there when you use?

Tony: He lives with his mom and older brother. We don't smoke if his mom is home, but she works so she is not home much.

Caregiver: What about his brother?

Tony: Him, oh sometimes he smokes with us. He is the one that got John started.

Caregiver: I knew it! What are you doing going over there when his mom is not home?

Therapist: Ms. Smith, I know this can be really hard for you to hear. Normally, it would make sense for you to try to correct Tony about this, yet when we are in these sessions it is important that Tony feels free to tell us what is really going on.

Caregiver: You mean I have to hear all of this and not be able to do anything?

Therapist: I know it must feel that way. Yet, if you think about it, you *are* doing something for

Tony, something that is very hard to do and requires a lot of work on your part. You have brought him here for treatment and you are doing your best to help him.

Caregiver: Okay, so what am I supposed to do?

Therapist: Listen to him, I'm asking you to be able to hear what Tony is saying about his drug use and to trust that you and I will be able to work together with Tony to come up with solutions that can help him.

Caregiver: Well, what do I do when I hear things that make me want to change what I am doing with Tony, like the rules in my house and who Tony can hang out with?

Therapist: That's good. I want you to have those thoughts. The reason you are here in treatment, rather than Tony and I working on this without you, is so that you can hear what Tony says, and together the two of us can help Tony decide how to deal with his triggers. After we know more about Tony's triggers and have done this ABC assessment, we will move on to developing plans to deal with each trigger. So one thing you can do, Ms. Smith, is to try and think of plans to help Tony deal with his triggers. We will make sure we write some of those plans down today before you leave if you like.

Tony: Great, you guys are getting all in my business. You are going to ruin everything.

Therapist: Tony, I know it seems like that, but your mom and I will work with you when we develop these plans. You'll be able to help decide what you should do.

Tony: So you are not gonna narc on John to his mom?

Therapist: We are focused on you, not John.

Tony: Okay, well, I can always stop doing this if I want.

Therapist: That's right, and we appreciate you sticking with it so far. Let's look at the form again. I want to make sure that I captured something you said on this sheet. You mentioned that John's older brother smokes with you sometimes.

Tony: Yeah, well, mostly he lets John smoke some of his stash. He doesn't really sit down with us.

Therapist: Okay, good to know. I can see how being at John's house is a trigger, especially when his brother is around. Ms. Smith, what do you think?

Caregiver: Yeah, I put John down as a person I thought Tony might be using with. It seems like being around John is a trigger as well as being at his house since he asks Tony to smoke with him.

Therapist: [to Tony and his caregiver] Those are two good examples of triggers for drug use. Please complete the rest of the form, and try to come up with at least two or three triggers for each question. There are also questions about people, places, and things that help you *not* to use drugs at the end of this form, and those are important. I am here if you need to ask questions. We will go over the form when you are done.

THERAPIST TASK 4.2: COMPLETING THE ABC ASSESSMENT

Therapist: [to Tony and his mother] Now we are going to learn the remaining parts of the ABC assessment. A few minutes ago, we found out about some of Tony's drug use triggers. Now we are going to look at what Tony does when those triggers happen and what the consequences of drug use are for him. I have a form that will help us keep all of this information organized;

it is called the *ABC Assessment* [Form 4.2]. Here is a copy. [Hands Tony and his mother each a copy of *ABC Assessment* (Form 4.2).]

Tony, now the easiest way to fill out this form is to have you think of the last time that you used a drug, and I will show you how to fill your response in on the form. Think of the last time that you used a drug or alcohol. Once you have a picture of that in your mind, tell me some things that may have triggered the use.

Tony: Last Friday I smoked a blunt at John's house. We always smoke on Fridays.

Therapist: Good, and so let's think about some of the triggers that you and your mom have been working on. What do you think may have triggered you to use drugs? Based on what you just said, I can write down "being with John," "being at John's house," and "Friday" since you often use on Friday.

Tony: I guess I was bored, so I called John. I knew he would have some pot.

Therapist: Okay, I will put boredom down in the trigger column here. Now please think about what thoughts and feelings you were having after experiencing boredom.

Tony: It would feel good to get high, and that I should celebrate since it was Friday.

Therapist: Okay, let me write those things down. So let me see—you were bored and it was Friday, time to celebrate—and that led you to think about getting high. It would feel good to get high. So what happened next?

Tony: I walked over to John's house, and Barry was there. We go over there because John's mom is usually gone in the afternoon. Between all of us, we rolled up a big blunt and smoked it in the backyard.

Therapist: Okay, good detail. This is the information we write down in the column marked "B" for "behavior." So you walked over to his house, Barry was there, his mom was not, and that led you guys to decide to use. So now, tell me what happened next.

Tony: We just smoked it.

Therapist: It will help if we have details. For example, who supplied the blunt? Where exactly did you go to smoke it? Did you have to do anything to get ready to smoke it?

Tony: Well, John pulled it out of his pocket. We walked behind this shed he has in his backyard, so his next door neighbor wouldn't see us. We can't smoke in the house or his mom will smell it when she gets home.

Therapist: Good detail. Anything else?

Tony: Well, I had matches that I carry for these kinds of times, so I pulled one out and lit it up.

Therapist: Okay, now let's look at the next column, marked "C" for consequences. Usually good things happen right after drug use—that is why people use. How did you feel?

Caregiver: Good things? How can you call smoking pot a good thing?

Therapist: Well, I have to agree that, from our perspective as adults, it is pretty hard to see the good side of a teenager using drugs. Especially if that teen is our child and we know how bad it can be for him. Yet people use drugs because they get something from it. They like it. So, to be able to help a person get off drugs, we have to understand what the drug is doing for them, how it helps them.

Caregiver: Okay, but I don't want Tony to think that anything good will come from his drug use.

Therapist: Tony, can you tell us how smoking made you feel better in some way?

Tony: I felt relaxed and kind of energized.

Therapist: What other good things happened?

Tony: I wasn't worrying about school or getting in trouble. I felt good.

Therapist: Now for the not-so-fun part. Can you think of some bad things that happened because of your use that afternoon?

Tony: Somehow my mom could tell that I was stoned when I went home. She got pretty upset and yelled at me.

Caregiver: You had red eyes and a dumb look on your face. It is easy to tell when you have been smoking grass.

Therapist: Ms. Smith, do you remember getting upset when Tony came home and you realized he was stoned?

Caregiver: I do, and I was so angry at him. I just can't believe he's still getting in trouble after everything we've been through. Then every time I have to yell at Tony, my husband and I get into it too.

Therapist: Tony, do you remember a fight between your mom and stepdad after your mom was upset with you for smoking?

Tony: Yes, it seems like every time I get in trouble everyone fights at home.

Therapist: That is a good observation, so let's look back over the form. Tony, do you have any questions about why we are doing this or about how to do it?

Tony: No.

Therapist: How about you, Ms. Smith?

Caregiver: No.

Therapist: Okay, for the next session I'd like Tony to come in with an *ABC Assessment* (Form 4.2) completed on one other drug use situation. Ms. Smith, it's your job to help Tony complete the form in the same way that I did. Tony, if you use drugs or alcohol between now and the next time we meet, go ahead and complete the form for those situations. If not, that's great and you can complete the form the same way but for not using. In that case, the behavior would be to "not use" and you would look at the ways you were able to avoid use. It's just as important to identify the people, places, and activities that surround you when you don't use as it is to identify those things that are around you when you do use. Fill out the form either way. I will be checking this when we meet next week.

Caregiver: When do we start to do something about these triggers?

Therapist: We start next week. We'll be developing plans, called self-management plans, to address the triggers of Tony's drug use.

Tony: Okay, so what if I run into triggers this week? What should I do?

Therapist: Well, if you like, we can take a few minutes now and discuss some triggers you are likely to run into and come up with some simple plans. Then next week we can evaluate them.

Caregiver: Good, I would like to do that.

Therapist: Okay, let's take 5 minutes to come up with some plans. The work you do this week may give us some ideas for your more detailed self-management plans next week.

[Therapist and family talk about some ways that Ms. Smith can help Tony avoid John over the next week and strategies Tony will try to use if he runs into John.]

CHAPTER 5

Self-Management Planning and Drug Refusal Skills Training

THERAPIST GOALS

1. **Help the youth and caregiver create a self-management plan—a template of the strategies and skills the youth and family will use to manage drug use triggers and contexts.**
2. **Teach the caregiver to aid the youth in implementing these strategies and to reinforce success.**
3. **Develop drug refusal skills for those drug use situations that are unavoidable.**

OVERVIEW OF SELF-MANAGEMENT PLANNING

Self-management planning is a process that helps youth to actively manage their drug use triggers and contexts. The therapist introduces self-management planning after it is clear that the caregiver and youth are able to conduct an ABC assessment. Self-management planning is a collection of strategies and skills designed to better manage each identified drug use trigger and situation. As with an ABC assessment, the self-management plan is revised continuously during treatment. The therapist helps the youth and caregiver review and modify the self-management strategies each session, paying special attention to times when the youth relapses or when new triggers for drug or non-drug use are identified.

In their successful treatment of drug-dependent adults with the CM approach, Budney and Higgins (1998) identified three basic ways of handling drug use triggers and situations.

1. *Avoid triggers and situations*—for example, take a different route home from school to avoid the home of a friend where drug use occurs.
2. *Rearrange the environment*—for example, get rid of items associated with triggers, such as pipes, bongs, rolling papers, and cigarette lighters.
3. *Make a new plan*—for example, develop different skills to cope with triggers and unavoidable contexts, and seek social support from non-drug-using peers.

Self-management planning should logically follow each ABC assessment. Thus, after every drug screen, whether the screen is dirty or clean, the therapist makes sure the youth and caregiver have completed an ABC assessment of the drug use or nonuse. Then the therapist, youth, and caregiver review aspects of the previous self-management plan that triggered drug use or helped the youth not to use drugs. The plan is then revised accordingly to help the youth with triggers that might be encountered in the coming week. In addition to avoiding drug use triggers, youth also need drug refusal skills and strategies for dealing with unavoidable social situations that increase the risk of drug use.

Drug refusal skills are a special subset of self-management strategies and are developed to assist the youth when he or she encounters unavoidable social situations that increase the risk of drug use. Most drug relapses in youth occur when they are with peers (Brown, Myers, Mott, & Vik, 1994) and while many negative peers can be avoided, it is impossible to predict and plan for all future situations. Hence, all youth receiving CM should work to create and practice a repertoire of tactics that they can access when faced with peer triggers. While drug refusal skills are particularly beneficial for use in unexpected situations, they also can be components of a self-management plan (e.g., having youth plan to utilize specific drug refusal skills to deal with social triggers). Therefore, developing effective skills for refusing drugs is crucial for long-term abstinence.

Aims and Time Frame of the Following Tasks

The primary treatment goals for this chapter are to help the youth and caregiver learn how to develop and practice strategies for dealing with common antecedents of the youth's drug use. Because youth drug use invariably occurs in social contexts, drug refusal skills are taught and practiced with each family as well. An experienced therapist working with a family that is engaged and actively participating will be able to introduce both tasks (i.e., self-management plans and drug refusal skills) for the first time in a single 1-hour session. Therapists with less experience or working with families requiring more time may prefer to set aside a separate 45- to 60-minute session for self-management planning and a 30- to 45-minute session for drug refusal skill training. Because drug refusal skills training can often be introduced in 30 minutes, therapists might prefer to tack this on to other CM introductory sessions that are short or end early such as the drug testing protocols (Chapter 7). Also, as noted previously, self-management planning and drug refusal skill training will become central to all CM sessions as treatment progresses.

THERAPIST TASK 5.1: DEVELOPING SELF-MANAGEMENT PLANS

Objectives

1. Help the youth and caregiver understand the rationale of self-management planning.
2. Coach the youth and caregiver in how to brainstorm plans to deal with triggers.
3. Teach the youth and caregiver how to weigh the costs and benefits of possible plans so they can choose the best possible strategy for dealing with triggers for drug use.
4. Have the youth practice a strategy for managing a drug use trigger during the session and ensure that the youth, with caregiver support, can practice the strategy between sessions.

Materials

- *Therapist Checklist 5.1: Self-Management Planning*
- *Self-Management Planning* (Form 5.1)
- *Self-Management Planning Example* (Handout 5.1)

Accomplishing the Objectives

Following the steps outlined in *Therapist Checklist 5.1: Self-Management Planning*, the therapist starts by introducing the concept of self-management planning with the youth and caregiver. The *Self-Management Planning Example* (Handout 5.1) can be used to help orient participants to the goals of this session. Therapist steps for completing self-management plans are outlined next.

Explain the Rationale of Self-Management Planning to the Youth and Caregiver.

The therapist explains that self-management planning is a process that uses specific strategies or plans to actively manage drug use triggers. Some of these strategies involve rearranging the environment so that the youth can avoid triggers for drug use, while others help the youth cope with triggers that cannot be avoided.

Brainstorm Plans to Deal with Triggers.

After reviewing the *Self-Management Planning Example* (Handout 5.1) with the family, the therapist hands the youth and caregiver each a blank *Self-Management Planning* worksheet (Form 5.1) and works with the family to determine an appropriate trigger to target in this exercise. Note that over time the therapist and family will develop strategies to deal with all of the triggers that seem to be contributing to or sustaining the youth's drug use. For the purposes of this first self-management session, it is helpful to pick a trigger that seems to play an important role in the youth's drug use and that the therapist feels can generate several potential plans from family members. The therapist writes the agreed-upon trigger in the appropriate space at the top of the form and then asks the youth and caregiver to brainstorm possible ways of dealing with that particular trigger. The therapist encourages the youth and caregiver to come up with as many solutions as possible and, as they are being generated, enters them in the left column of the form. It is important that the therapist and family focus on producing as many ideas as possible, without judging them or discussing whether they are feasible at this point in the session.

Note that experts in social problem-solving skills interventions for youth have found that the following principles help make brainstorming sessions effective (D'Zurilla & Nezu, 1999):

- *Quantity of solutions.* When coming up with ideas about solutions, *quantity* is important. The more ideas people have for solutions, the better.
- *Variety of solutions.* The greater the variety of solutions, the better.
- *Suspension of judgment.* Everyone should *suspend judgment* about the ideas for solutions while brainstorming.

The therapist might want to introduce these concepts to the youth and caregiver prior to asking them to generate solutions.

Select the Best Plan.

After the youth and caregiver have generated a list of potential strategies to manage the identified trigger, the therapist shifts the focus of the session to help them decide which strategy should be implemented. Selecting the best solution is essentially a cost–benefit analysis. Going down the list of plans, the therapist first asks the family to think about what the benefits of using that particular approach might be. Next, the therapist and family discuss what costs or barriers the plan would entail. The benefits the youth lists should be positive outcomes he or she feels might be accomplished in the immediate future by following the plan; for example, keeping his or her mind off drugs, staying busy, feeling physically and psychologically better, staying focused in school, making someone who is important to the youth happy, or decreasing arguments with parents. Costs that youth commonly report include embarrassment, being viewed poorly by the peer group, losing important relationships (e.g., boyfriend or girlfriend, other friends), feeling left out, being bored, and having to make new friends or develop new skills.

After the benefits and costs to using each plan have been listed, the therapist and family talk about how hard it will be for the youth to carry out each strategy. Then, using a scale from 1 to 10 (where 1 = easy and 10 = extremely difficult or unrealistic), the youth rates each strategy based on his or her perceptions of how hard it would be to follow that plan. Finally, the youth and family decide which plan or plans the youth will attempt to use the following week when presented with that particular trigger. Optimally, strategies that have relatively low costs but high benefits should be chosen. For instance, in the

Self-Management Planning Example (Handout 5.1), the youth would most likely choose to try plan C—*Walk Tiffany, my girlfriend, to classes as a way to avoid Mike*—because this plan appears to be beneficial, seems realistic, and is rated as easiest by the youth. Note that the therapist will likely want to predict that Tiffany might not always be available and so help the youth pick a backup plan to practice and have in reserve should it be needed.

Early in the development of self-management skills, the therapist should help the youth select a strategy that is relatively easy to carry out. Accordingly, the practice, feedback, and real-life testing of strategies described next should first focus on triggers that are relatively common. For example, if seeing a drug-using peer in the school hallway is a relatively common event, and avoiding the peer by going down a different hall is rated by the youth as a fairly easy strategy, then this trigger and management strategy might be the focus of self-management sessions early in treatment. As the youth demonstrates the ability in sessions and real-life tests to manage the triggers that are more commonplace with strategies that are fairly easy to implement (like avoiding the youth in the hall), the therapist should begin to include triggers that are less commonplace and to practice management strategies rated by the youth as more difficult in role plays and real-life situations. The ultimate goal is to build the youth and family's skills so that the youth has the capacity to effectively implement a self-management strategy in response to a trigger, whether the strategy is easy or hard and whether the trigger is commonplace (e.g., peer in hallway) or less frequent (e.g., being at a party with drug users).

Practice Self-Management Plans.

After a relatively easy strategy has been selected, the therapist creates opportunities for the youth to practice using the tactics. This practice begins with the therapist or caregiver modeling the strategy. Then the therapist sets up role plays that more closely reflect the situation described by the youth. For example, the therapist and caregiver might act in the same way as a drug-using peer or girlfriend acts to trigger the youth's substance use. The therapist should make sure that the youth has practiced the plan and received specific feedback (described next) several times before trying the tactic in real-life situations.

The therapist takes the following steps when helping the youth and caregiver practice the strategy:

- Model the strategy in session.
- Role-play the strategy in session.
- Provide specific feedback about what the youth did well during the role play and about things he or she might need to do differently for the strategy to be effective.
- Repeat steps 2 (role-play) and 3 (provide specific feedback), enlisting the caregiver's help in providing feedback. The therapist might need to coach caregivers on how to make specific statements about what the youth did well and what needs to be improved.
- Plan a real-life test of the strategy the next time the situation arises.

This process of modeling, role playing, providing feedback, and planning a real-life test of a self-management strategy is repeated for strategies rated as more difficult as treatment progresses. In going through these steps, the therapist should ensure that the youth understands what was good about what he or she did in the role play and why he or she might need to do some things differently. The feedback must be highly specific to enable the youth to master the skills and strategies needed to manage the triggers effectively.

After the therapist, youth, and caregiver concur that the youth has had sufficient practice to try the strategy in a real-life situation, the therapist asks the youth to implement the strategy the next time a real-life opportunity arises. The therapist also provides feedback as soon as possible after the youth has tried the strategy in the real-life situation.

THERAPIST TASK 5.2: DEVELOPING DRUG REFUSAL SKILLS

Objectives

1. Help the youth develop drug refusal skills to use during unavoidable social situations that increase the risk of drug use.
2. Help the youth develop a drug refusal style that is likely to be effective in his or her social context.
3. Provide opportunities through role plays for the youth to practice using drug refusal skills to manage drug offers in unavoidable social situations.
4. Teach the caregiver to assist the youth in this process.

Materials

- *Therapist Checklist 5.2: Developing Drug Refusal Skills*
- *Social Network Information* (Form 5.2)
- *Drug Refusal Skills* (Form 5.3)
- *Drug Refusal Skills Example* (Handout 5.2)

Accomplishing the Objectives

Following the steps outlined in *Therapist Checklist 5.2: Developing Drug Refusal Skills*, the therapist starts by introducing the broad concept of drug refusal skills to the youth and caregiver and describes the importance of these tactics in both obtaining and sustaining abstinence. The *Drug Refusal Skills Example* (Handout 5.2) can be used to help orient participants to the goals of this session. A summary of the steps to be followed to help youth create individualized drug refusal skills is outlined next.

Gather Information about the Youth's Social Network.

Drug refusal skills are more likely to be effective if they are developed to fit the unique context of the youth's peer network and social context. A *Social Network Information* worksheet (Form 5.2) is provided to assist the therapist and caregiver in better understanding the youth's peers. First, the therapist asks the youth and caregiver to name some friends with whom the youth likes to socialize. Then, following the outline of the form, the therapist tries to assess some of the qualities of the youth's peer group such as their background, group activities, and the youth's status in the group. Next, the youth is asked to identify assertive drug refusal behaviors that his or her peer group would accept or to think of a friend who is assertive, looked up to by peers, and drug free. Behaviors exhibited by a socially adept peer can provide examples of drug refusal behaviors that are likely to be successful (e.g., "The judge is having me tested every week and will send me away if I have another dirty screen"). The therapist reminds the youth to think about what type of body language, eye contact, tone of voice, and facial expressions might need to be exhibited to be successful with his or her peer group.

Brainstorm Drug Refusal Strategies.

After the therapist has collected sufficient information about the social context in which the youth uses drugs, the work can shift to helping the youth and caregiver develop drug refusal strategies for the youth to implement in this peer context. A *Drug Refusal Skills* worksheet (Form 5.3) and an example (*Drug Refusal Skills Example* [Handout 5.2]) are provided to assist with this process. These strategies and their respective forms mirror the approach taken with self-management planning. The steps to follow include:

- Identify a recent situation involving the youth's peer group or another social context in which the youth accepted an offer to use drugs. List this situation in the box at the top of the page labeled "Situation."
- Generate potential strategies or methods for saying "no" with the youth and list these in the spaces provided on the form. To facilitate this process, the participants should:
  - Consider the *antecedents* to the drug use situation and any *thoughts* and *feelings* the youth had during the time leading up to drug use, as specified in the ABC assessment. This information can assist in understanding, for example, the youth's fears in refusing drugs from a peer or irrational thoughts related to accepting or refusing drugs.
  - Guide the youth in identifying as many drug refusal strategies as possible (brainstorming) and list these strategies in the left column of Form 5.3.
  - If the youth is having difficulty generating realistic plans, share drug refusal strategies that other adolescents have found to be effective in similar situations (see Troubleshooting Tips section in this chapter for examples).
  - Use information generated during the discussion of the youth's social network

to help develop strategies that are likely to make sense given the youth's peer group.

Guide the Youth in Selecting Drug Refusal Strategies.

This process mirrors the steps taken in the self-management planning process. Utilizing the *Drug Refusal Skills* (Form 5.3) worksheet, the youth should be asked to generate a list of the possible benefits and costs of each proposed strategy. The difficulty of each strategy should then be rated on a scale from 1 (easy) to 10 (most difficult). The youth should then select the strategy or strategies he or she would like to attempt to implement. As with self-management plans, the youth should be encouraged to select a tactic that he or she feels has strong benefits and few costs and is fairly easy to carry out.

Practice the Selected Drug Refusal Skills.

The therapist then works with the youth to model and role-play the selected strategies. To make this process as realistic as possible, the therapist should try to enlist caregivers or other family members, especially those who know the peers, to serve as "actors." Remember that different strategies are effective for different youth, so be enthusiastic in modeling and role-playing each strategy with the youth and family. Caregiver participation in this process can be very beneficial, because it can help parents learn how to coach their child in this process while also facilitating their understanding of the peer struggles the youth might be facing.

Provide Feedback.

With the youth and family members, identify effective components of the strategies as well as those that might need to be adjusted to increase effectiveness. Role-play these new strategies until the youth is comfortable with the strategies he or she plans to use. The therapist might need to coach the caregiver or family members on how to provide appropriate feedback regarding the youth's performance on the task.

TROUBLESHOOTING TIPS

Objective

The purpose of this section is to help therapists anticipate common challenges to conducting self-management planning and drug refusal skills training and to suggest strategies to address these difficulties.

Challenges and Solutions

Youth and Caregiver Have Difficulty Generating Ways of Managing Triggers and Developing Drug Refusal Plans.

The therapist provides strategies based on his or her own clinical experiences and the experiences of colleagues who are using CM with other youth confronted with similar triggers and social contexts. Examples of commonly used drug refusal strategies include (1) telling friends the truth and asking for help; (2) pretending to be sick or to have a medical condition that precludes use; (3) using sports or the desire to be in other activities that require being straight; (4) wanting to avoid serious consequences from parents, probation, or other authority figures; and (5) wanting to earn privileges that require clean screens.

Lack of Community Resources and Prosocial Activities to Facilitate Implementation of Self-Management Plan.

The therapist works with the youth and caregiver to identify sources of social support—extended family, friends, and neighbors—that can help provide resources needed to facilitate the youth's access to prosocial activities. For example, social supports might need to be enlisted to help provide a ride to an after-school program or to help with a registration fee for a prosocial activity. As described in the Troubleshooting Tips for Family Engagement Difficulties section of Chapter 3, the therapist might need to work with youth and caregivers to help them identify informal (e.g., family members, relatives, colleagues, friends) and formal (e.g., recreation center programs; church-, mosque-, or synagogue-based programs; activities sponsored by civic clubs) sources of support to facilitate the youth's access to positive activities. The therapist should become familiar with the range of resources in the community that might be available to youth and families. The therapist or agency might need to obtain discounted rates and scholarships for youth and families to help supplement treatment.

Intense Drug Cravings Interfere with Implementation of Self-Management Plan and Drug Refusal Skills.

The youth with a long-standing history of substance abuse might have drug cravings as he or she stops using drugs. The cravings can intensify as the youth responds to triggers with new skills that prevent drug use. When cravings intensify, the youth is more likely to relapse. The self-management plan for a youth who experiences drug cravings should include strategies for managing these cravings. Strategies that therapists can introduce to help the youth manage cravings include:

- Relaxation training.
- Thought-stopping techniques.
- Habit reversal training (i.e., practicing a competing response).

Descriptions of the implementation of these strategies are beyond the scope of this book. However, *The Relaxation & Stress Reduction Workbook* (Davis, Eshelman, & McKay, 2000) might be a helpful tool for therapists who want to learn more about these therapeutic techniques.

THERAPIST CHECKLISTS, FORMS, AND HANDOUT FOR CHAPTER 5: SELF-MANAGEMENT PLANNING AND DRUG REFUSAL SKILLS TRAINING

THERAPIST CHECKLIST 5.1

Self-Management Planning

Case number: ______________ **Session date:** ______________

I have explained that (check each item covered in session):

___ *Self-management planning* is the process of identifying specific strategies that will help (*youth's name*) manage drug use triggers.

___ *Self-management planning* occurs each time a drug use or non-use trigger is identified in an ABC assessment.

___ (*Youth's name*), (*caregiver's name*), and I will work together to develop plans to help (*youth's name*) avoid triggers.

___ We will work together to help (*youth's name*) come up with ways to rearrange his/her environment to avoid triggers.

___ We will also both work to develop strategies or plans to help (*youth's name*) cope with triggers that cannot be avoided.

I have given the youth a copy of the *Self-Management Planning* worksheet (Form 5.1) and have:

___ Guided youth and caregiver in identifying a trigger for the youth's most recent drug use event.

___ Provided and reviewed *Self-Management Planning Example* (Handout 5.1) to facilitate the process.

___ Helped the youth and caregiver brainstorm how to avoid or manage the trigger.

___ Recorded plans to avoid or manage the trigger in the "Plan" column.

___ Helped the youth and caregiver identify benefits and costs for each plan.

___ Recorded benefits and costs for each plan in the "Cost–Benefit Analysis" column.

___ Instructed the youth to rate the difficulty of each plan in the "Difficulty" column.

___ Assisted the youth and caregiver in selecting a plan or plans.

___ Modeled the chosen role play.

___ Helped the youth and caregiver role-play the chosen plan(s).

___ Provided constructive feedback on the role play.

(cont.)

___ Included the caregiver in role-play exercises and provided feedback about the youth's implementation of the plan.

___ Repeated the sequence described above with other identified triggers.

___ Asked the youth to attempt the chosen plan(s) for next week.

___ Clarified and addressed any confusion or concerns expressed by the youth and caregiver.

THERAPIST CHECKLIST 5.2

Developing Drug Refusal Skills

Case number: ______________ **Session date:** ______________

I have explained that (check each item covered in session):

___ Situations that involve being around people and friends or acquaintances (social situations) can be full of triggers for drug use. Often when people slip up or use drugs again, the slipup had something to do with a social situation, such as being asked by a friend to use.

___ Even though some drug use triggers can be avoided, no one is able to avoid all social situations that can tempt them to use drugs. Therefore, learning ways to tell people "no" or developing "drug refusal skills" is an important part of getting clean and staying clean.

___ In order to better help [youth's name] identify skills that will be effective, we will first need to find out more about his/her current friends (peers) and their social networks.

I have given the youth and caregiver a copy of the *Drug Refusal Skills* worksheet (Form 5.3) and have:

___ Used the *Social Network Information* worksheet (Form 5.2) to gather information about (*youth's name's*) friends, his or her relationships, and how his or her social network seems to work.

___ Brainstormed potential drug refusal skills with (*youth's name*) and (*caregiver's name*):

- ☐ Identified situations in which the youth has accepted offers to use drugs.
- ☐ Generated drug refusal skills for each situation.
  - ☐ Considered information gathered about the youth's social network.
  - ☐ Considered antecedents, thoughts, and feelings experienced by the youth during the time leading up to drug use.
  - ☐ Shared drug refusal strategies used effectively by other youth in similar situations.

___ Recorded all potential skills/strategies on the *Drug Refusal Skills* worksheet (Form 5.3).

___ Helped the youth and caregiver identify the benefits and costs for each skill/strategy.

___ Recorded benefits and costs for each skill/strategy in the "Cost–Benefit Analysis" column.

___ Instructed the youth to rate the difficulty (1–10 scale) of each plan in the "Difficulty" column.

___ Assisted the youth and caregiver in selecting a plan or plans.

___ Modeled and role-played potential drug refusal skills identified.

(cont.)

___ Guided the youth in selecting those skills he/she could use effectively.

___ Practiced the selected skills through role-play exercises.

___ Provided constructive feedback on the role-play performance.

___ Included the caregiver in the process of identifying skills, conducting role plays, and providing feedback about implementation of the selected skills.

___ Repeated these steps for other situations in which drug offers might be unavoidable.

FORM 5.1

Self-Management Planning

Name: ______________________ **Date:** __________

Drug of choice: ______________________

Trigger:

Use this form to help create ways to manage the triggers of your drug use. This will help reduce the chances that triggers will lead to drug use. **Fill out one form for each trigger.**

Plan	**Cost–benefit analysis** *Benefits*	*Costs*	**Difficulty** (1–10 scale; 10 = most difficult)
A)			
B)			

(cont.)

Plan	**Cost–benefit analysis** *Benefits*	 *Costs*	**Difficulty** (1–10 scale; 10 = most difficult)
C)			
D)			
E)			
F)			

FORM 5.2

Social Network Information

List of Friends:

Status in Peer Group:

Where in the hierarchy of the peer group does the youth stand (e.g., leader of the pack, initiates activities, influences others in the group, follows along with the group's decisions, activities)?

What is the youth's role in the peer group (e.g., risk taker, leader of the group, follower, "clown")?

Group Activities:

What kinds of activities does the group engage in? Are some activities favored more than others?

(cont.)

Peer Background Information:

Are peers on probation or involved in criminal activity? Are they out of school or in school? Are they drug using or nonusing? Does the youth have any prosocial peers?

Acceptable Assertive Behaviors:

Who are some of the assertive peers in the group? Describe them. Do they use a certain tone of voice, facial expressions, or body language? Do they follow through with what they say? How do others respond to them?

Identify a peer who is "looked up to" by other peers; describe him/her. What is his/her "style"?

Identify peers who are drug free. How do they interact in the group successfully while still avoiding drug use? What specific things do they say or do to avoid using?

FORM 5.3

Drug Refusal Skills

Name: ______________________ **Date:** ____________

Situation:

Potential strategies for saying "no"	**Cost–benefit analysis**		**Difficulty** (1–10 scale; 10 = most difficult)
	Benefits	*Costs*	
A)			
B)			

(cont.)

Potential strategies for saying "no"	**Cost–benefit analysis** *Benefits*	*Costs*	**Difficulty** (1–10 scale; 10 = most difficult)
C)			
D)			
E)			

HANDOUT 5.1

Self-Management Planning Example

Name: John B. **Date:** 10/5/11

Drug of choice: Marijuana

Trigger:

Seeing friend Mike in the halls at school—asks me to skip class and go smoke

Use this form to help create ways to manage the triggers of your drug use. This will help reduce the chances that triggers will lead to drug use. **Fill out one form for each trigger.**

	Cost–benefit analysis		**Difficulty** (1–10 scale; 10 = most difficult)
Plan	*Benefits*	*Costs*	
A) Talk to Mike ahead of time and let him know I am in this program where I get in trouble for using pot. Tell him my probation officer is saying he will send me to jail if I get caught.	Mike might stop trying to get me to smoke with him.	Mike might think I'm a loser for not smoking. He may tease me.	5
B) Figure out the times I usually run into Mike in the hallway and find a different route during those times.	Avoid the trigger.	I might still run into him.	3

(cont.)

Self-Management Planning Example *(page 2 of 2)*

Plan	Cost–benefit analysis *Benefits*	 *Costs*	**Difficulty** (1–10 scale; 10 = most difficult)
C) Walk Tiffany, my girlfriend, to classes as a way to avoid Mike since they do not get along and he does not talk to me when I am with her.	Avoid the trigger, make Tiffany happy, keeps my mind off drugs.	I might feel left out from what my friends are doing.	2
D) Switch my classes from "A-block" to "B-block." Most of my friends who use drugs are in "A-block" with me.	Really easy to avoid bad friends, and I have some good friends in "B-block" who do not use.	I would not see my best friends or Tiffany very much. The guys would start leaving me out of things. Tiffany may get another guy.	8
E)			
F)			

HANDOUT 5.2

Drug Refusal Skills Example

Name: Joanne **Date:** 5/12

Situation:
My friends (Rick, Tanisha, Shelly) ask me to smoke with them after the ball game on Friday nights

Potential strategies for saying "no"	**Cost–benefit analysis** *Benefits*	*Costs*	**Difficulty** (1–10 scale; 10 = most difficult)
A) Talk to all of them ahead of time and tell them I am getting drug tested and cannot use because I don't want to get in trouble with my parents.	They might understand and not ask me to smoke with them. Tanisha is most likely to help me say "no."	They might try and get me to take something to cheat the drug test. Shelly cheated her drug test before and she did not get caught.	6
B) Tell them I don't feel good and want to go home.	Easy to do, they won't want me to give them germs. It is easy for me to fake being sick.	This will probably only work once. After that they will know I am lying.	2

(cont.)

Potential strategies for saying "no"	**Cost–benefit analysis** *Benefits*	*Costs*	**Difficulty** (1–10 scale; 10 = most difficult)
C) Tell them I am trying out for the basketball team and can't be on the team if I get caught using. Smoking makes my asthma worse so I need to quit for now so I can play better.	They might buy this because they know I really want to make the team.	I'll miss hanging with them on Friday nights. They will have all of that fun without me. I will feel left out at school on Mondays.	3
D) Tell them that my parents are paying me to watch my little brother, so I have to go home and don't have time to use.	They will probably think I am telling the truth.	They will still think I should use a little with them before I go home.	4
E)			

Sample Dialogues: Self-Management Planning and Drug Refusal Skills Training

INTRODUCTION TO SELF-MANAGEMENT PLANNING

Therapist: [to Tony and his mother] Today, we are going to learn how to take the ABC assessment information we have been working on and use it to help Tony come up with plans to avoid drug use.

First, let's look over the *Self-Management Planning Example* [Handout 5.1] and the *Self-Management Planning* worksheet [Form 5.1] that I am passing out. It will be easiest to understand how to complete this sheet if we think about an actual trigger that Tony recently experienced or that has been difficult for him.

Based on the work you have been doing on triggers, what triggers are causing you the most problems?

Tony: I don't know.

Caregiver: Well, I've noticed that John is almost always around when Tony uses drugs. Don't you think he might be a trigger for you?

Tony: Yeah, I guess so.

Therapist: Okay, so I'm going to write his name down here in this box at the top of the page. Now, when do you see John?

Tony: Well, since he was expelled from school, I mostly see him after school. I usually walk by his house on the way home.

Therapist: Good. Now I would like for both of you [Tony and Ms. Smith] to try and think of strategies that Tony can use to deal with the fact that seeing John is a trigger for drug use. Try not to worry about whether your ideas are good or not. Just give me any thoughts that come into your head and I will write them down. We call this part brainstorming, and we are just trying to get a bunch of ideas right now.

Tony: Well, I guess I could go home another way.

Therapist: Good. What else?

Tony: I could get my mom to pick me up after school.

Caregiver: You know I am too busy.

Therapist: Ms. Smith, let's just put down as many ideas as possible right now. We can figure out which are the best in a few minutes.

Tony: I could go to basketball practice instead of walking home.

[Session continues as more ideas are generated.]

Therapist: That's good. Now, let's look more closely at each of these plans. Your first idea was to go home a different way. What are the benefits of doing that?

Tony: Well, it would be easy for me to do and there is another way home that is actually shorter.

Therapist: What are the downsides of this plan?

Tony: Well, at first it would probably work and be no problem. After awhile, Tony would probably come and try to find me.

Caregiver: Yeah, he would probably call Tony on his cell phone after a day or two.

Therapist: Your cell phone?

Tony: Yeah, that's how he usually gets me.

Therapist: Good point. I am going to put "cell phone" down in the trigger space on another *Self-Management Planning* worksheet [Form 5.1]. We will get to that one next. For now, let's get back to ways to avoid John after school.

Caregiver: We were talking about Tony's plan to avoid John by taking another way home.

Therapist: Is that a plan that you can really do?

Tony: Yeah, there's a shortcut I can take that will avoid John's house. I could do it.

Therapist: How hard would that be, on a scale from 1 to 10, with 1 being easy and 10 being very hard?

Tony: About a 2 or 3.

Therapist: Okay, let me write that down. Now, the second idea was for you to have your mom pick you up after school. Can you do that, Ms. Smith?

Caregiver: Not really. I have to work until 5:00 P.M. and he gets out of school at 3:00 P.M.

Therapist: Benefits?

Tony: It would work. I would avoid John.

Caregiver: Until he calls you.

Therapist: Yes, we will need to deal with the phone trigger. Ms. Smith, it sounds like we should rate this idea as a 9–10 on our difficulty scale because it not very possible.

Caregiver: I agree.

Therapist: Tony, how about the next plan, to go to basketball practice?

Tony: The problem with that one is that practice doesn't start for 3 more weeks. The benefits are that I think it would be a lot easier to avoid John if I was playing basketball.

Therapist: When it does start, how many days a week, and how long will it last?

Tony: It'll go till 5:30 or 6:00 P.M. I think we will practice 5 days a week after school.

Caregiver: I could pick him up on those days, after practice. Tony, are you sure you can make the team?

Tony: Yeah, there are a bunch of open spots this year, and I'm better than two guys who made it last year.

Therapist: Great, so it sounds like Tony can go to practice every day after school in about 3 weeks. That should really help you to avoid John. Tony, how hard will that be? Any problems we have not thought about?

Tony: It'll be easy.

Therapist: So, it seems that for now, we've settled on the first plan. You will take the shortcut and avoid John's house. When basketball starts, that will take up your time and you can avoid John that way. That brings me to the cell phone. It looks like we should problem solve around that trigger too. I am going to put "cell phone" down in the trigger space on another *Self-Management Planning* worksheet (Form 5.1).

Tony: No, I really need my phone.

Therapist: First, do you agree that it is a trigger?

Caregiver: I know it is. He is always calling his friends on it. I can never tell who he is talking to.

Therapist: Okay, let's brainstorm on some things we can do to help with that trigger. The main idea is that we don't want John to be able to call him because that may trigger drug use.

Tony: I don't know.

Therapist: Well, some of my other clients have had the number blocked, or given it a different ringtone, or even turned their phone off and used their message box to screen calls.

Tony: I could give him a different ringtone.

Therapist: Okay, I will put that down for the first plan. What is another plan?

Tony: I could turn the phone off and check my messages.

Therapist: Okay, what else?

Caregiver: He could let me hold the phone for a few weeks.

Tony: Ah man, I need my phone.

Caregiver: I could let you use it certain times. I could screen your calls.

[Note: Therapist, caregiver, and Tony follow the same procedures to complete the *Self-Management Planning* worksheet (Form 5.1) concerning the cell phone trigger. They end up with a plan in which Tony will change the ringtone for John's calls. They agree that they can try different options in subsequent weeks if this first, easiest plan is not effective.]

Therapist: [to Tony and Ms. Smith] I'd like you to attempt the plans we've written down on this sheet for next week. We'll talk about how things turned out during our next session. I predict good things next week. Also, we need to figure out how you can get in touch with me soon after Tony has tried a plan. That way Tony knows he is not alone and we are trying to help him. Why don't I call you guys about 5:30 P.M. on Monday? That way, we can find out how the plans are working before we meet again.

INTRODUCTION TO DRUG REFUSAL SKILLS TRAINING

Therapist: Tony and Ms. Smith, out of all the strategies we have been creating for Tony's self-management plan, I think that Tony having to tell his friend John that he doesn't want to use drugs with him is going to be one of the harder things for Tony to do. Tony, what do you think?

Tony: I don't know.

Therapist: Well, no matter how much we plan to help you avoid the trigger of seeing John, sooner or later you're probably going to run into him and he may offer you drugs.

Caregiver: Yes, and you are going to have to tell him you don't want to use drugs.

Therapist: So I'd like to work with you both on how to handle this situation.

Tony: Okay.

Therapist: First, I have some forms to give you (*Drug Refusal Skills* worksheet [Form 5.3], *Drug Refusal Skills Example* [Handout 5.2]). These are similar to the ones we used to create self-management plans during our last session.

Tony: You really like forms.

Therapist: Yeah, helps me stay organized. Now, let's get started. Tony, tell me the last situation you can remember in which John offered you drugs.

Tony: I ran into John on the way home from school about 2 weeks ago, and he asked me to smoke a blunt with him.

Therapist: Okay, I will put "running into John after school" in the box labeled "Situation." Now what might you do and say the next time you run into John that would help you avoid using drugs?

Tony: I can tell him I don't want to use because my mom, stepdad, and therapist are on my back and checking me with urine screens.

Therapist: Okay, I will write that in the first box of the left column. What else might you do?

Tony: I don't know. I think the plan I just mentioned will work.

Therapist: Some of the other young men I've worked with who like to play sports have told their friends they don't want to use because it will hurt their athletic skills or it may get them kicked off the team.

Tony: Yeah, that might work. I could say I can't smoke because of trying to make the basketball team.

Caregiver: Tony could just tell John the truth. He could say that he is trying to quit and ask John to go away.

Therapist: Sure, I'll write that down too.

[Session continues as more ideas are generated.]

Therapist: Okay, now let's think about the strengths and barriers to each of these ideas and rate each one on how difficult it may be to do.

[Session continues as plans are evaluated.]

Therapist: Out of all these things we talked about, which strategy do you think may work for you?

Tony: I can tell John that I don't want to use because I am playing basketball, and it will hurt my game.

Therapist: Great. Let's do role play together, and I want you to tell me that you don't use because you are starting to play basketball again. I am going to pretend to be John and that I ran into you on the street. I am going to offer you drugs, and I want you to refuse me. Ms. Smith, I'd like for you to watch us closely and see if we are doing a good job of imitating this interaction with John. You can also see if you have ideas that may help Tony.

Caregiver: Okay, I'll try.

Therapist, playing John: Tony, hey, where have you been?

Tony: I've been around, just chilling.

Therapist, playing John: Cool. I have a blunt. Let's go smoke.

Tony: Man, I can't. I'm playing basketball now and it will mess up my game.

Therapist, playing John: For real? Why are you punking out on me like that?

Tony: It ain't even like that. Man, you know I ain't no whiz kid; B-ball is my only shot of getting out of this place.

Therapist, playing John: All right, I hear you. So what—you're not going to hang out with me now?

Tony: No man, you are my boy! I want to hang with you. I just can't smoke. How about you come with me to a pick-up game on Saturday at the rec center? My stepdad will be at the game. He'll buy lunch for us.

Therapist, playing John: All right, I'll see you there.

Therapist: Tony, I thought you did a good job. I especially liked how you said that you weren't going to accept the offer, and that you looked me straight in the eye when you told me. Ms. Smith, how did that look?

Caregiver: Pretty good. I think John might go for that.

Therapist: Let's role-play another situation.

[Session continues as more ideas are role-played.]

CHAPTER 6

The Point-and-Level Reward System

THERAPIST GOALS

1. **Explain and sign a CM contract with the youth and caregiver.**
2. **Develop a reward menu with the family that specifies what the youth will earn with clean drug screens and alcohol breath scans.**
3. **Teach the youth and caregiver how to implement the point-and-level reward system.**

OVERVIEW OF THE POINT-AND-LEVEL REWARD SYSTEM

The purpose of the CM point-and-level reward system is to provide incentives for clean drug screens and alcohol breath scans and disincentives for dirty screens or scans. The point-and-level reward system is presented in the form of a contract that is signed by the youth, caregiver, and therapist. Next, a reward menu that clearly specifies what the youth can purchase with earned points is developed. Essentially, the point-and-level system provides incentives for the youth not to use drugs and disincentives for using drugs. When a youth has not used drugs and tests clean, he or she is rewarded with points that can be exchanged for various rewards or for access to important privileges provided by caregivers as outlined in the reward menu. Conversely, drug use is punished by the loss of points and valued privileges. Youth and caregivers are taught to track points earned using a system that simulates a checking account.

To arrange the point-and-level reward system, the therapist conducts these tasks:

1. Signs a contract with the youth and caregivers that lays out the rules by which the youth will earn, lose, and spend points.
2. Develops an individualized reward menu with the family that identifies positive

items and social activities or privileges that the youth can earn by providing clean urine drug screens and alcohol breath scans.

3. Sets up and monitors a checkbook system for tracking points earned, spent, or lost.

Completing the Contract

A standardized contract has been developed (*Point-and-Level System Contract for Youth and Caregiver* [Form 6.1]) for use with all youth who have a caregiver or supportive adult involved with their treatment (see Chapter 9 for a contract designed for use when no adult supports are available). This contract outlines the rules of the point-and-level reward system and sets the stage for the family to work with the therapist to develop a reward menu. Because the contract is somewhat complicated, *Point-and-Level System at a Glance* (Handout 6.1) helps clarify the levels of treatment and points earned at each level.

Developing the Reward Menu

The reward menu is generated by the youth, family, and therapist immediately after the contract is signed and is vital to ensuring that the terms of the contract are meaningful and motivating for the youth. Because each reward menu must be individualized, therapists and family members expend substantial effort generating a list of potential rewards, evaluating the appropriateness of the rewards, vetting them with both the youth and caregivers, and finally assigning points to the rewards and placing them on the reward menu. The reward menu is then consulted after each drug test, and points and privileges are administered or withheld on the basis of the results of the youth's drug screen and breath scan.

Types of Rewards

Therapists providing CM might have access to incentives in the form of vouchers or gift resources that can be used to help motivate youth to achieve sobriety. When available, these incentives can facilitate the effective implementation of CM. Yet it is important for therapists to also help families find indigenous family- and community-based resources to reward youth abstinence as well. This chapter provides information on how to implement the point-and-level system both with and without the use of vouchers or gift rewards that are external to the family's ecology.

Keeping Track of Points Earned and Spent with the Checkbook System

Finally, families are taught to carefully track the points earned by their child. An accounting system modeled after the banking practice of using checks and checkbooks is demonstrated. This method of tracking points is often appealing to adolescents and targets developmentally appropriate skill acquisition.

Aims and Time Frame of the Following Tasks

The primary goal of the interventions outlined in this chapter is to help the family create a well-specified behavioral plan that will encourage and facilitate the youth's drug abstinence. This is accomplished in three steps, which include signing a contract, creating a reward menu, and tracking the points earned and spent. The first step of reviewing and signing the contract is often accomplished in 30 minutes or less. The next step is more complex, and many therapists need an hour or more to develop a well-specified reward menu. The third step, reviewing the point tracking system, often takes approximately 30 minutes to complete. One potential strategy is to complete these three tasks in two 60-minute sessions. Another is to give the family members homework and ask them to complete some forms prior to the session (e.g., completing a *List of Potential Rewards* [Form 6.2]). Many therapists prefer to schedule a 90-minute session to accomplish the majority of these tasks.

THERAPIST TASK 6.1: INTRODUCING THE POINT-AND-LEVEL REWARD SYSTEM AND CONTRACT

Objectives

1. Discuss the goals, rationale, and contract format of the CM point-and-level system.
2. Review *Point-and-Level System at a Glance* (Handout 6.1), and read the *Point-and-Level System Contract for Youth and Caregiver* (Form 6.1) with the family.
3. Obtain signatures on the *Point-and-Level System Contract for Youth and Caregiver* (Form 6.1).

Materials

- *Therapist Checklist 6.1: Introducing the Point-and-Level System and Contract*
- *Point-and-Level System at a Glance* (Handout 6.1)
- *Point-and-Level System Contract for Youth and Caregiver* (Form 6.1)

Accomplishing the Objectives

Following the steps outlined in *Therapist Checklist 6.1: Introducing Point-and-Level System and Contract*, the therapist hands each family member a copy of the contract (*Point-and-Level System Contract for Youth and Caregiver* [Form 6.1]) and *Point-and-Level System at a Glance* (Handout 6.1). The checklist contains useful phrasing that can help set the tone for treatment—suggesting that getting free from drugs and alcohol might be conceptualized as a full-time job and that the contract and reward system are much like an agreement the youth would have with an employer concerning payment for work accomplished. This contract might help the family reframe their thoughts about the youth's drug use and establish a collaborative tone in working together to assist the youth. The contract is designed to be read to the family, and the handout helps to clarify the details. This task is complete when the contract has been read and signed by the participants.

THERAPIST TASK 6.2: COMPLETING A REWARD MENU

Objectives

1. Explain to youth and caregiver that potential rewards might include items, activities, and privileges.
2. Meet individually with youth to:
   a. Develop first draft of *List of Potential Rewards* (Form 6.2).
   b. Identify rewards that might serve as a "most valued privilege," or MVP.
   c. Assign possible point values to suggested rewards.
3. Meet individually with caregivers to:
   a. Complete *List of Potential Rewards* (Form 6.2).
   b. Edit *List of Potential Rewards* (Form 6.2).
   c. Determine the MVP.
   d. Transfer appropriate rewards and MVP to *Reward Menu* (Form 6.3).
   e. Assign final points to rewards on *Reward Menu* (Form 6.3).
   f. Review the *Reward Menu* (Form 6.3) for completeness.
4. Confirm and finalize *Reward Menu* (Form 6.3) with the youth and caregiver together.

Materials

- *Therapist Checklist 6.2: Completing a Reward Menu*
- *List of Potential Rewards* (Form 6.2)
- *Reward Menu* (Form 6.3)
- *List of Potential Rewards Example* (Handout 6.2)
- *Reward Menu Example* (Handout 6.3)

Accomplishing the Objectives

Following the steps outlined in *Therapist Checklist 6.2: Completing a Reward Menu*, the therapist starts by handing each family member a blank *List of Potential Rewards* (Form 6.2) and *Reward Menu* (Form 6.3). It is often helpful to also distribute the corresponding examples (*List of Potential Rewards Example* [Handout 6.2] and *Reward Menu Example* [Handout 6.3]) so that participants can better understand the goals of the session. Therapist steps for completing a reward menu with the family are outlined next.

Explain Rewards to the Youth and Caregiver.

The therapist explains that the goal of this session is to help the family create a reward menu that outlines what the youth will earn with clean drug screens and alcohol breath scans. This reward menu is going to play a very important role in treatment because it will be used to help motivate the youth to get clean and stay clean. The therapist might also explain that everyone is different, and so what is rewarding for one person might not be rewarding for another. One of the best ways to find out what motivates or rewards youth is to see what they spend their time doing, or what they try to do whenever they get a chance. Hence, the family and therapist will go over some forms to try and better understand what kinds of activities, privileges, and things the youth would like to purchase with points earned from clean screens. The *List of Potential Rewards* (Form 6.2) describes some categories of items, privileges, and activities that many adolescents find rewarding.

Often the therapist will find it easier to get youth to open up about what they would like to earn without their parents in the room to judge or comment. The therapist can ask the caregiver to leave the session at this point and start to complete the *List of Potential Rewards* (Form 6.2) with the youth alone. It is certainly appropriate, however, to keep the youth and caregiver together for this part of the exercise if they can work with the therapist to accomplish the tasks effectively.

Develop List of Rewards with the Youth.

Using the *List of Potential Rewards* (Form 6.2), the therapist works with the youth to try and determine what types of rewards he or she is currently receiving and what items, privileges, and activities he or she would like to earn (see *List of Potential Rewards Example* [Handout 6.2]). The therapist tries to help the youth identify reasonable rewards that can be provided by the caregiver. If the therapist has access to vouchers or gift certificates, items that can be purchased with the vouchers may also be incorporated into the reward list. With parental approval, these will ultimately be placed on the *Reward Menu* (Form 6.3) and used as rewards for staying clean. Once the *List of Potential Rewards* (Form 6.2) has been completed, the therapist reviews it with the youth to select a potential MVP. Selecting an appropriate MVP is crucial because the youth will only be able to access the MVP when his or her screens and scans are clean. Hence, the MVP should be an item that (1) the youth values highly and (2) the caregiver can withhold or give on the basis of each drug screen. Examples of powerful MVPs include cell phone, computer, or video game use and access to transportation. The therapist also tries to get a sense of how important each of the various rewards are for the youth, because the goal is ultimately to have the *Reward Menu* (Form 6.3) contain items that the youth values.

At this point in the session, the therapist may ask the youth to leave and bring the caregiver in to complete the next steps. This separation of participants makes it easier for the therapist to empower the caregiver to take ownership of the behavioral plan that is being developed in the form of a reward menu. Also, although the youth's input is important, the caregiver has the final say about what rewards can be earned by the youth. Hence, the session might move faster and be easier to manage if the youth is not in the room. It is certainly appropriate, however, to keep the youth and caregiver together for this part of the exercise if they can work with the therapist to accomplish the tasks without hindering the process.

Meet with the Caregiver to Modify List of Potential Rewards (Form 6.2) and Convert This to a Reward Menu (Form 6.3).

During the individual meeting with the youth's caregiver, the therapist completes the following tasks.

Complete the *List of Potential Rewards* (Form 6.2). The therapist helps the caregivers understand that the rewards list is an important method for identifying the kinds of replacement rewards that can successfully compete with current reinforcers that maintain the adolescent's drug use. By making sure the youth gets the identified replacement rewards when he or she is not using drugs, as evidenced by clean screens, the caregivers can help the youth to stop using drugs. Using the *List of Potential Rewards* (Form 6.2) that was partially completed with the youth previously, the therapist helps the caregivers to review all of the privileges the youth currently receives or might like to receive. Often caregivers are not fully aware of privileges their child is already receiving (e.g., extra clothes, video games, special snacks or meals), and one of the goals of this step is to help them understand that they have the ability to provide a number of important low-cost rewards for their adolescent. Caregivers might also realize that they have been inadvertently rewarding their child by giving him or her access to privileges despite drug use and other irresponsible behaviors.

Edit the *List of Potential Rewards* (Form 6.2). This is a crucial step in the process of developing a functional reward menu. Using the *List of Potential Rewards* completed by the youth, the therapist helps the caregiver determine which privileges are appropriate for the youth to earn. As a rule of thumb, each reward should meet the following criteria:

- The reward does not contribute to irresponsible behavior such as drug use. For example, the youth should not be able to earn unsupervised time with drug-using peers or be allowed to purchase items like posters or video games with content that is known to trigger drug use.
- The reward is not an essential activity (e.g., participation in school sports or religious youth group) that is good for the youth and should be provided regardless of drug screen results.
- The caregiver is willing and able to withhold the privilege if it is not earned.
- The privilege or reward is reasonable given the context in which the youth and caregiver live.

Determine the MVP. Next, the therapist helps the caregiver identify a privilege that the youth values from the edited list of potential rewards, providing the caregiver information about the youth's requested MVP. Good candidates for the MVP are privileges the youth values and that the caregiver knows the youth will work hard to get and will be disappointed to lose. Importantly, the MVP needs to be a privilege the caregiver can provide or withhold weekly depending on the results of each drug screen. Note that youth who abuse drugs with a shorter half-life, such as cocaine, which are excreted from the body in less than a week will require more frequent drug screens. As a result, the MVP attached to these screens may need to be given or withheld more frequently depending on the screen result. Examples of privileges that might be good candidates for MVPs include access to video games, cell phone use, time with friends, and transportation. Note that the MVP should be tailored to the youth's interests.

Transfer Appropriate Rewards and MVP to the *Reward Menu* (Form 6.3). After the caregiver and therapist have agreed on an appropriate list of rewards and the MVP, these are then written down on a blank copy of the *Reward Menu* (Form 6.3) (also see *Reward Menu Example* [Handout 6.3]). If the therapist is helping to subsidize rewards through vouchers or gift certificates, care should be taken to ensure that at least half of the rewards are being provided by the caregiver, family, or other individuals in the youth's natural ecology. This is an important step. The vouchers are meant to help the therapist and family members get youths motivated and started in treatment, yet the odds of the youth being successful in achieving abstinence are greatly enhanced when caregivers are able to learn to control and deliver these rewards and consequences within their own natural ecology.

Assign Final Points to Rewards on *Reward Menu* (Form 6.3). Next, the therapist helps the caregiver determine a point or value for each reward (except for the MVP, which is always given if the drug screen is clean or withheld if dirty). One rule of thumb is to assign a lower number of points for items or privileges that are easy for the caregiver to provide or afford on a daily basis and a greater number of points for privileges that can be provided only weekly or monthly. A privilege the caregiver feels can easily be provided daily would be worth 1 point, a privilege or item the caregiver feels could be delivered weekly might be worth 7 points, and a privilege or item given monthly would be worth 30 points. For example, having a caregiver pack the youth's lunch might be worth 1 point, renting a movie might be worth 5 to 7 points, and allowing a friend to spend the night might be worth 15 to 20 points (see also *Reward Menu Example* [Handout 6.3]).

Review the *Reward Menu* (Form 6.3) for Completeness. After the therapist and caregiver have completed a draft of the *Reward Menu* (Form 6.3), it is reviewed for several key components.

Quick Check of Reward Menu (Form 6.3)

- The *Reward Menu* (Form 6.3) should contain the youth's MVP at the top. The MVP should be a privilege that can be used to support drug abstinence. ***The MVP is not assigned a point value because it will be given or taken away with each drug screen or breath scan based on the results of that test.***

- The *Reward Menu* (Form 6.3) should be *very simple* and contain a list of items or privileges that the caregiver and the youth agree are reinforcing for the youth and are provided by the caregiver or therapist (e.g., vouchers). These entries should have assigned point values based on how reinforcing they are to the youth and how costly they are to the caregiver.
- If the therapist is subsidizing youth rewards with vouchers or gift certificates, at least half of the items on the *Reward Menu* (Form 6.3) should be rewards the caregiver plans to provide.
- The *Reward Menu* (Form 6.3) *might* (this is not required) also include *a list of rewards* that the youth is willing to work for as privileges for appropriate performance in other domains of life that are being addressed in treatment (e.g., school attendance, meeting curfew, associating with socially appropriate peers). These privileges should be clearly separate from those being provided or withheld for drug abstinence or use. In other words, privileges the youth can earn for clean screens should not overlap with items that the therapist and caregiver might need to withhold for other problem behaviors.

Confirm and Finalize Reward Menu (Form 6.3) with the Youth and Caregiver Together.

After completing the individual meeting with the youth and finalizing the draft of the *Reward Menu* (Form 6.3) with the caregiver, the therapist and caregiver then meet with the youth and review the outcomes of their meeting. The therapist is careful both to convey enthusiasm to the youth about the list of rewards finalized by the caregiver and to encourage the youth to voice any concerns with the outcome. The caregiver, not the youth, ultimately determines the rewards. Yet if real discrepancies exist between what the youth wants and what the caregiver is willing to provide, then further sessions might be needed to develop a consensus that is acceptable to both parties. Otherwise, the youth might not be motivated to get clean.

THERAPIST TASK 6.3: MONITORING POINTS EARNED AND EXCHANGED WITH THE CHECKBOOK SYSTEM

Objectives

1. Teach the youth and caregiver how to keep track of points earned and spent by the youth as part of his or her contingency contract.
2. Teach the youth checkbook-keeping skills.

Materials

- *Therapist Checklist 6.3: Monitoring Points Earned and Exchanged with the Checkbook System*
- *Point-and-Level System at a Glance* (Handout 6.1)

- *Checkbook* (Form 6.4)
- *Personal Checks* (Form 6.5)
- *Checkbook Example* (Handout 6.4)
- *Personal Checks Example* (Handout 6.5)

Accomplishing the Objectives

The therapist starts by handing each family member a copy of the checkbook and check forms used to track points (*Checkbook* [Form 6.4], *Personal Checks* [Form 6.5]), and the examples of correctly completed forms (*Checkbook Example* [Handout 6.4], *Personal Checks Example* [Handout 6.5]). The therapist may also provide clients with another copy of *Point-and-Level System at a Glance* (Handout 6.1), which concisely summarizes the rules of the point-and-level system. The next steps are closely outlined in *Therapist Checklist 6.3: Monitoring Points Earned and Exchanged with the Checkbook System.* The therapist might find it helpful to read this checklist to the family. To summarize, the therapist reminds the family of the rules of the point-and-level system and describes how the points will be tracked using the *Checkbook* (Form 6.4). The youth is then taught how to write *Personal Checks* (Form 6.5), and the family is encouraged to use this system. The therapist is careful to keep a copy of all points earned and exchanged in the client's chart as well, because families might forget to bring their checkbook to the next treatment session.

TROUBLESHOOTING TIPS

Objective

The purpose of this section is to help therapists anticipate common challenges to explaining the contract, developing the reward menu, and teaching families to track the youth's points as they are earned and spent.

Challenges and Solutions

Caregivers Do Not Believe That Children Should Be Rewarded for Abstaining from Drug Use.

The therapist might want to start by agreeing with the caregiver that we should not have to "pay" youth to not break the law. Similarly, the therapist can concur that the perspective of the caregiver is, in fact, reasonable. In so doing, the therapist is starting "where the caregiver is," an important step to engagement. The therapist might then explain that, from a purely practical perspective, the youth is in a situation in which he or she is experiencing serious difficulties; otherwise, the child would not be in treatment for a drug problem. The therapist might convey the bottom line that (1) something needs to be done quickly to decrease the youth's drug use and (2) CM has a strong track record in reducing youth substance use. The following points can be emphasized in addressing the caregiver's concern:

- The strategy of providing rewards for abstinence will be used only during times of great need to help get the youth on a more productive path.
- The therapist and caregiver will work together during the course of treatment to help the adolescent develop more intrinsically rewarding pursuits (e.g., success in school, work, and extracurricular activities).

A second strategy is to suggest to the caregiver that the youth's problems, including substance abuse, are so serious that the child's primary job now is to stop using drugs. In this scenario, the therapist emphasizes the following points:

- In general, people are expected to work hard and to try to get their work done when they are on the job. So, just like in any job, hard work should be rewarded.
- The youth's participation in this program might also help to prepare him or her for the work world by reinforcing responsible behavior and teaching skills such as keeping and balancing a checkbook. That is, the youth will be learning more life skills than just staying away from drugs.

The Family Has Few Resources to Use as Rewards and Privileges.

When caregivers have concerns about their lack of resources to provide desired rewards and privileges, the therapist might emphasize that he or she will help the family identify and access adequate resources throughout the course of treatment. The therapist should be familiar with community resources for prosocial activities such as recreation centers, churches, mosques, or synagogues and civic organizations that sponsor youth activities. In addition, the therapist might help the family identify resources within their own social support system. There are different types of social support (e.g., favors, advice, emotional support, loans), and therapists can help caregivers identify people in their lives who provide these types of support. For information concerning helping caregivers access indigenous social supports, please see Caregivers Have Limited Social Supports discussion in the Troubleshooting Tips for Family Engagement Difficulties section of Chapter 3.

Additionally, sometimes caregivers think they do not have the resources to provide rewards because the rewards will be too costly. The therapist should be prepared to give concrete examples of affordable activities and rewards. For example, a favorite meal or free time can be rewards if they are enjoyed by the youth, and these types of rewards are far less expensive than video games and iPods. The *List of Potential Rewards* (Form 6.2) is designed to help caregivers realize that youth often receive many small privileges throughout the day that can be earned (i.e., snacks, free time, transportation) rather than simply given regardless of behavior. Also, caregivers often underestimate the importance of a very valuable, yet inexpensive resource: their time. Adolescents need and desire caregivers' company and supervision, both of which can be very reinforcing. Caregivers might need help from the therapist to better understand what they can do with their child and how to go about making this activity reinforcing. Examples include cooking a meal together, going to a park or shopping center, fishing, working on a project, watching a movie or sporting event, or finding time to talk about things that are important to the youth. With some creative guidance, most youth and caregivers should be able to agree on some realistic and inexpensive rewards that the youth would like to earn.

The Checkbook System Is Too Difficult for Youth or Caregivers to Use.

If the checkbook system proves too complicated or cumbersome, therapists can shift to a simple poster or chart to monitor the accumulation and spending of points.

Family and Therapist Have Difficulty Picking Out an Effective MVP.

Helping family members decide on an appropriate MVP is an important part of CM. An effective MVP should be:

- Something the youth really wants to obtain.
- Something the youth really does not want to lose.
- Something the caregivers can easily give or withdraw with each drug screen and breath scan.
- Something the youth cannot easily attain from other sources.

Some examples of MVPs that have been successfully used by families include:

- Cell phone usage—youths should have access to the cell phone only when they are compliant with the most recent drug screen request and the screen is clean. If a youth tests dirty, it is recommended the cell phone be removed until the next clean screen. Weekly screens should be in place to ensure the phone continues to be earned. If the youth avoids or skips a screen, it is considered dirty and the phone should be removed until a clean screen is obtained.
- Access to favorite clothes, shoes, makeup, hair care products, or jewelry—some caregivers lock up all favorite shoes, clothes, or other items, leaving only essentials, and allow access to these favorites only when the youth's most recent screen is clean.
- Use of music player—some youth already have an iPod or MP3 player and are motivated to be able to use them. Again, care should be taken to ensure that the youth has access to the player only when he or she is compliant with drug screening and has recently tested clean.
- Use of video or computer games—like music players, access to electronic games can be a powerful motivator. Caregivers find that this privilege works best when access to the game player or computer is cut off until the youth has a clean screen. Some families find it helpful to remove plug-in cords and hand-held remotes or keyboards from the house with each dirty result, replacing the items only when

the youth tests clean. Caregivers might need to store the essential electronic parts at their workplace or other secure place unknown to the youth, such as the trunk of their car or a neighbor's house.

- Access to transportation—many youth are highly motivated to have access to the family car, to be driven places, or to be given subway, bus, or train passes. Care should be taken to specify exactly what is earned and to ensure that it is withheld until a recent clean screen is documented.
- Time spent with caregivers doing something the youth wants to do—some youth respond well to caregivers doing something special for them each time they are clean. Ideas should be generated by the family and might include, for example, preparing a favorite meal together, renting a movie of the youth's choice, or allowing the youth to skip some routine chores or tasks he or she finds unpleasant.

It is important for therapists to check in routinely with families to ensure that the MVP in place is being delivered appropriately and seems to be working. Therapists often find it necessary to change or modify the MVP several times during the course of treatment.

Substance Screens Remain Dirty or the Youth Remains Noncompliant.

The youth might continue to have dirty screens even when he or she has lost the MVP or failed to earn points despite excellent ABC assessments of drug use and strong self-management plans. Alternatively, the youth might be noncompliant with all aspects of the treatment plan. In either case, if the primary treatment goals are not being met, the therapist should consider the introduction of graduated sanctions.

Rationale for Graduated Sanctions. Most youth continue to engage in problem behavior, including drug use, because the costs of doing so do not outweigh the benefits. Therefore, an increasingly aversive set of sanctions is developed to shift the cost–benefit ratio in favor of desired behavior, including abstinence from drug use.

When to Consider Using Graduated Sanctions. Therapists should consider using graduated sanctions when either of the following occur: 2 consecutive weeks of dirty screens (longer if the youth was a chronic substance abuser) or 2 consecutive weeks of noncompliance with drug treatment. The success of graduated sanctions depends largely on the ability of the youth's caregivers to start and maintain the sanctions. Implementing sanctions can be both emotionally and physically difficult for caregivers, because the youth is expected to resist the sanctions with all of his or her abilities. Caregivers, with problem-solving and emotional support from the therapists, will need to hold fast in the face of youth attempts to stop the sanctions plan. Given the centrality of caregivers to the success of graduated sanctions, it will not be possible to implement graduated sanctions with a youth who does not have caregivers involved in treatment. Thus, therapists are advised not to attempt graduated sanctions when the drug treatment protocol is being implemented in individual therapy with the youth only (i.e., permanent caregiver absence from treatment).

Components of Graduated Sanctions. As described previously, a youth who tests dirty or refuses to be tested during the course of treatment (1) does not receive points for that screen and (2) loses his or her MVP until abstinence is demonstrated with clean screens. The loss of the MVP is actually the first step on the stairway of graduated sanctions, and this step (along with the ABC assessment and self-management planning described in previous chapters) will often be all that is needed to decrease youth substance use. If, however, the youth's substance use or noncompliance with treatment continues, a second level of sanctions might include loss of other privileges the youth currently receives and values (e.g., access to friends, TV, video games) until he or she tests clean. If the youth's drug screens remain dirty, sanctions can escalate to include the continued loss of existing privileges (i.e., restricted to home and school), extra chores at home (i.e., washing car, cleaning house), or community service (i.e., helping at the Salvation Army, cleaning a neighbor's yard).

When Graduated Sanctions Are Ineffective. If the caregivers are implementing the sanctions as specified in treatment sessions with the therapist and a youth's substance screens continue to be dirty for 4 to 6 consecutive weeks, the therapist and caregivers together should consider the possibility that additional treatment resources might be needed to effectively manage the youth's drug use. The therapist should review the American Society of Addiction Medicine Patient Placement Criteria to determine whether the youth might benefit from referral to a service that can provide more intensive care.

Challenges Specific to Clinicians Using Vouchers or Gift Certificates

The Youth Cashes In Points Only for Vouchers, Ignoring Family-Based Rewards.

This is a common problem because the therapist voucher rewards are often more expensive and readily appealing to adolescents. Although voucher rewards provided by therapists are designed to grab the youth's interest and help motivate him or her to have clean screens, the family-based rewards are an essential part of treatment. When family-based rewards are not being cashed in by the adolescent, the therapist should consider taking one or several of the following steps:

- Review the *List of Potential Rewards* (Form 6.2) carefully with the youth and caregiver. The goal of this review is to better assess what things the caregiver and others in the youth's ecology can do with him or her that might be reinforcing.
- Revise the *Reward Menu* (Form 6.3) to include items that the youth wants that are provided by people in the youth's context.
- Check to ensure that the *Reward Menu* (Form 6.3) has appropriate points assigned to family-based rewards.
- Increase the cost, in points, for voucher awards.
- If the *Reward Menu* (Form 6.3) appears to have adequate family-based

reinforcements that are appropriately priced, consider giving the youth 5 bonus points with the next clean screen but require that he or she spend these on a family-based reward.

- Ultimately, the contract might need to be revised with the youth and caregiver to require that some percentage of points (i.e., 50%) be spent on family-based rewards.
- Consider revising the total amount of voucher dollars available for the youth. There should not be enough vouchers to subsidize more than half of the youth's treatment. Clinicians in our studies have had limits of 100 to 150 voucher dollars per youth.

The Youth Runs Out of Voucher Money before Treatment Is Complete.

This scenario is likely to occur if family-based rewards are not well integrated into the point-and-level system or if the youth takes a long time to gain 10 straight weeks of abstinence. In either case, the youth should not be allowed to earn more than the agreed amount of vouchers from the therapist. The family and therapist will need to find indigenous rewards to place in the *Reward Menu* (Form 6.3) when the vouchers are depleted.

THERAPIST CHECKLISTS, FORMS, AND HANDOUTS FOR CHAPTER 6: THE POINT-AND-LEVEL REWARD SYSTEM

THERAPIST CHECKLIST 6.1

Introducing the Point-and-Level System and Contract

Case number: ______________ **Session date:** ______________

I have explained that (check each item covered in session):

___ This contract is a very important part of CM treatment and is going to serve as an agreement between us, like an agreement you might have with the person or company you work for.

___ Often getting off drugs/alcohol can be like working a full-time job.

___ This contract will outline some things that we (*caregiver and therapist*) will be able to provide for you, (*youth's name*), when you have clean urine drug screens/breath scans.

___ This contract also describes about how your family can help you, (*youth's name*), as you learn to get clean from drugs.

___ Here is a copy of the contract [hand out copy of *Point-and-Level System Contract for Youth and Caregiver* (Form 6.1)]. Please read along with me, and I will explain as we go.

___ Here is a sheet that describes the point-and-level system more concisely. I will go over this with you after we read the contract [hand out copy of *Point-and-Level System at a Glance* (Handout 6.1)].

___ We may need to revise or change this contract as we go through treatment. If changes are needed, we will all work on them together like we are doing now.

___ [Answer questions concerning the point-and-level system. *Point-and-Level System at a Glance* (Handout 6.1) might be used as a tool.]

___ [Read and sign contract with youth and caregiver.]

I have:

___ Provided a copy of the *Point-and-Level System Contract for Youth and Caregiver* (Form 6.1) to the youth and caregiver.

___ Obtained signatures that youth and caregiver agree to participate.

___ Put a copy of the signed contract in the client's chart.

THERAPIST CHECKLIST 6.2

Completing a Reward Menu

Case number: ______________ **Session date:** ______________

I have explained that (check each item covered in session):

Step 1: Explain Concept of Rewards to the Youth and Caregiver

___ Now that we have a contract, it is time to determine how (*youth's name*) would like to be paid for the hard work he/she is going to do to stay off drugs and alcohol.

___ We need to come up with some things that (*youth's name*) can earn that (*caregiver's name*) or the family can provide.

___ *If vouchers are being provided*: (*Youth's name*) will be able to spend some of the points he/she earns in this program to buy rewards that I will provide in the form of vouchers/gift certificates. [Provide details of rules concerning vouchers.]

___ The reason we are coming up with these rewards is that we know it can be very hard to stop using drugs and alcohol, so we are trying to find things that will help motivate (*youth's name*) and that will compete with drug and alcohol use.

___ Here is a form [give client and caregiver a copy of *List of Potential Rewards* (Form 6.2)] we will use to identify what rewards and privileges (*youth's name*) is already getting from your family and what else he/she might want to earn.

___ (*Caregiver's name*), I am going to start by going over this form with (*youth's name*) to see what sorts of rewards he/she would like to earn. Next, I will meet with you to modify this form, and then we will all get back together and agree on a final reward menu.

Step 2: Develop List of Potential Rewards with the Youth

___ [Complete *List of Potential Rewards* (Form 6.2) with youth.]

___ Now, let's look at this list and pick out one or two things to be your most valued privilege (MVP). The MVP needs to be something that really motivates you to stay away from drug and alcohol use, as well as something that your caregiver can provide every time that you have a clean screen. [Go over list and pick out two to three potential MVPs.]

___ Next, I'd like for us to look at the things you would like to get as rewards and think about how many points each item should cost. In general, little things that you could earn from your caregiver about once a day (like talking on the phone or staying up later) should cost around 1 to 2 points, while things that you could earn once a week, like going to the movies, should cost about 7 points. [If vouchers are being provided, specify the dollar value of each point. For instance, the cost of vouchers might be set at 1 dollar a point.]

___ Now, I am going to meet with your caregiver and go over this same list. After that, we'll get back together with you and finalize the list of things you can earn for being clean.

(cont.)

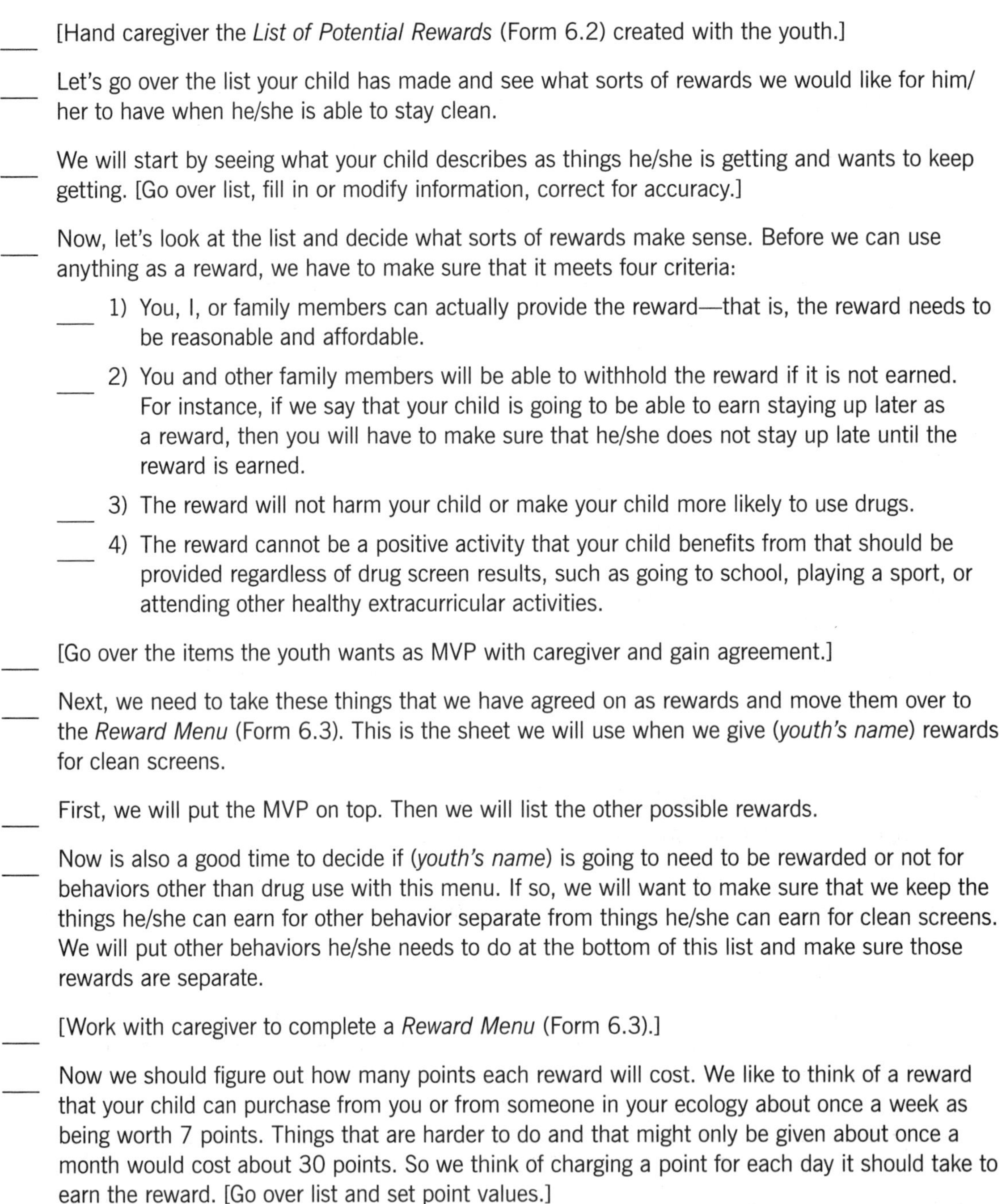

Step 3: Create *Reward Menu* (Form 6.3) with Caregiver

___ [Hand caregiver the *List of Potential Rewards* (Form 6.2) created with the youth.]

___ Let's go over the list your child has made and see what sorts of rewards we would like for him/her to have when he/she is able to stay clean.

___ We will start by seeing what your child describes as things he/she is getting and wants to keep getting. [Go over list, fill in or modify information, correct for accuracy.]

___ Now, let's look at the list and decide what sorts of rewards make sense. Before we can use anything as a reward, we have to make sure that it meets four criteria:

- ___ 1) You, I, or family members can actually provide the reward—that is, the reward needs to be reasonable and affordable.
- ___ 2) You and other family members will be able to withhold the reward if it is not earned. For instance, if we say that your child is going to be able to earn staying up later as a reward, then you will have to make sure that he/she does not stay up late until the reward is earned.
- ___ 3) The reward will not harm your child or make your child more likely to use drugs.
- ___ 4) The reward cannot be a positive activity that your child benefits from that should be provided regardless of drug screen results, such as going to school, playing a sport, or attending other healthy extracurricular activities.

___ [Go over the items the youth wants as MVP with caregiver and gain agreement.]

___ Next, we need to take these things that we have agreed on as rewards and move them over to the *Reward Menu* (Form 6.3). This is the sheet we will use when we give (*youth's name*) rewards for clean screens.

___ First, we will put the MVP on top. Then we will list the other possible rewards.

___ Now is also a good time to decide if (*youth's name*) is going to need to be rewarded or not for behaviors other than drug use with this menu. If so, we will want to make sure that we keep the things he/she can earn for other behavior separate from things he/she can earn for clean screens. We will put other behaviors he/she needs to do at the bottom of this list and make sure those rewards are separate.

___ [Work with caregiver to complete a *Reward Menu* (Form 6.3).]

___ Now we should figure out how many points each reward will cost. We like to think of a reward that your child can purchase from you or from someone in your ecology about once a week as being worth 7 points. Things that are harder to do and that might only be given about once a month would cost about 30 points. So we think of charging a point for each day it should take to earn the reward. [Go over list and set point values.]

(cont.)

___ Now, let's go back over the *Reward Menu* (Form 6.3) briefly again to make sure that we have it all. I have a checklist here:

☐ MVP is at the top and does not cost points.

☐ All other items that are rewards for abstinence from drugs (except MVP) have points assigned to them.

☐ If some of the nontherapist, family-based rewards are going to be used for behaviors other than abstinence, these are on a separate page or at the bottom of the page.

☐ The rewards for nonabstinence behaviors (like school attendance) do not overlap with rewards for abstinence.

If vouchers/gift certificates are provided by the therapist:

☐ At least half of the rewards are for items that the caregiver/family provides. In other words, no more than half of the rewards come from therapist vouchers.

☐ The dollar/point value is set. For instance, each point is worth 1 dollar.

___ Now it is time to bring your child back in and go over the *Reward Menu* (Form 6.3) with him/her.

Step 4: Confirm and Finalize the *Reward Menu* (Form 6.3) with the Youth and Caregiver

___ [Meet with the youth and caregiver and go over the *Reward Menu* (Form 6.3), including the MVP and points assigned, and modify as needed to get joint youth–caregiver buy-in.]

THERAPIST CHECKLIST 6.3

Monitoring Points Earned and Exchanged with the Checkbook System

Case number: ______________ **Session date:** ______________

I have explained that (check each item covered in session):

___ Next, we will go over how to track the points that (*youth's name*) earns.

___ We are going to use a checkbook system. [Give copies of *Checkbook* (Form 6.4), *Checkbook Example* (Handout 6.4), *Personal Checks* (Form 6.5), and *Personal Checks Example* (Handout 6.5) to the youth and caregiver and have them review *Point-and-Level System at a Glance* (Handout 6.1).]

___ I am going to record 25 points in the *Checkbook* (Form 6.4) as a bonus for starting CM.

___ During the first part of treatment, while (*youth's name*) is in Level I, we will record 12 points every week that he/she has a clean drug screen or breath scan.

___ If (*youth's name*) has more than one screen or scan a week, we will divide the 12 points so that they add up to 12 if all the screens/scans are clean. For example, if we give two screens a week, each is worth 6 points.

___ If the screen or scan is dirty, we will record 0 points.

___ After (*youth's name*) has been clean for 6 weeks *in a row*, he/she will move to up to Level II.

___ In Level II, (*youth's name*) will earn 24 points for each week his/her screens are clean.

___ (*Youth's name*) may spend points when his/her most recent drug screen and breath scan are clean and when he/she has not missed or refused any screens or scans. Remember that a missed screen or scan is considered "dirty."

___ (*Youth's name*) may only spend the points he/she has. That is, she/he may not go into debt or have the balance go below zero.

___ When (*youth's name*) spends points, he/she will write a check and we will complete the checkbook balance forms, just like a real checking account.

___ In other words, when (*youth's name*) writes a check, the transaction should be dated and the number of points spent should be recorded under the payment/debit column and subtracted from the balance.

___ We will both (family and therapist) keep a copy of the checkbook balance sheet.

___ Let's go over the example sheets. [Review examples in Handouts 6.4 and 6.5 with family.]

FORM 6.1

Point-and-Level System Contract for Youth and Caregiver

We have agreed that helping you stop using drugs/alcohol is a very important job that needs to be done. This contract will help outline what each of our roles will be in that work. It describes a plan by which you can earn points and privileges as rewards when you have clean urine screens and alcohol breath scans each week. You can trade in your points to your caregiver for rewards and privileges that we agree on. You will also earn a most valued privilege (MVP) from your caregiver each time that you have clean screens.

Now, here's more information about the point system (also see *Point-and-Level System at a Glance* (Handout 6.1]):

Level I (from start of treatment until 6 straight weeks of clean screens):

- You will receive 25 points today for starting the program. This will happen only once.
- Points can be traded for rewards.
- We will create a list of rewards you would like to earn, called a reward menu.
- Rewards can be activities (e.g., movies), things (e.g., clothes), or privileges (e.g., use of car).
- A urine drug screen will be conducted at least once a week, maybe more often. Alcohol breath scans will be conducted whenever your caregiver or therapist thinks you might have been drinking.
- You will earn 12 points per week for clean urine drug screens and alcohol breath scans.
- If the drug screen and breath scan are negative (clean), you will be able to cash in some earned points for rewards.
- You will also get something called a most valued privilege, or MVP, from your caregiver each time you have a clean urine screen and alcohol breath scan.
- We will work together to decide on an MVP that will help motivate you to stay clean.
- If the drug screen or breath scan is positive (dirty), then:
  - You will not earn points.
  - You will not earn your MVP until you test clean again.
  - You will not be able to purchase rewards until you test clean again.
- You will keep track of your points with a checkbook and write checks to your caregiver or therapist to cash in points.
- You may only spend points when your most recent drug screen was clean.
- You may only spend points that you have already earned. In other words, you cannot go into debt in your checkbook or spend points you have not yet earned.

Level II (after 6 straight weeks of clean screens):

- When you have been clean for 6 weeks in a row, you will advance to Level II.
- In Level II, you will earn a total of 24 points (12 bonus points) for each week your screens are clean.
- Just like in Level I, you will earn your MVP and be able to write checks to spend points for rewards when your screens and scans are clean.
- If you have a dirty urine screen or breath scan while you are in Level II, you will drop back to Level I.
- You will have to test clean for 4 more weeks in a row to earn your way back to Level II again.

(cont.)

Level III (after 4 straight weeks of clean screens in Level II)

- Once you have tested clean for 4 weeks in a row at Level II, you will advance to Level III.
- In Level III, you will work with your therapist and caregivers to figure out how to help you have continued success staying drug and alcohol free.
- You will develop a sobriety maintenance plan, which is a plan for you and your family to help you stay clean in the future. This plan will likely include drug testing at high-risk times and family-based rewards for abstinence.

Your signature means that you agree to participate in this program.

______________________		______________________	
Youth	Date	Caregiver	Date
Therapist	Date	Caregiver	Date

FORM 6.2

List of Potential Rewards

Type of reward	What I get	What I want	What caregiver provides
Transportation			
Clothing			
Favorite dessert/snack			
Meals			
Laundry			
TV use			
Curfew			
Have a friend visit			
Invite friend for sleepover			

(cont.)

Type of reward	**What I get**	**What I want**	**What caregiver provides**
Non-drug/alcohol party/ get-together			
Privacy time			
Trips with family/friends			
Car (use, ownership, registration, insurance, payments)			
Phone (use, minutes, payments)			
Computer (use, minutes, Internet)			
Weights, sports equipment			
Music player/iPod			
Play sports			
Other item:			
Other item:			

FORM 6.3

Reward Menu

Rewards/Privileges	Cost
	Rewards for Drug Abstinence

Rewards for Responsible Behavior in Other Domains (optional)

FORM 6.4

Checkbook

Name: ______________________________

Record all deposits or payments that affect your account.

Date	Description of transaction	Deposit/ Credit (+)		Payment/ Debit (–)		Balance	

FORM 6.5

Personal Checks

Date ____________________

PAY TO THE ORDER OF ____

____ POINTS [ ]

FOR ____________________ ______________________________

Date ____________________

PAY TO THE ORDER OF ____

____ POINTS [ ]

FOR ____________________ ______________________________

HANDOUT 6.1

Point-and-Level System at a Glance

	Level I	Level II	Level III
Clean screen	1. Start with 25 points 2. Earn 12 points per week 3. Earn MVP[a] 4. Points can buy incentives from the reward menu 5. a. First time in Level I: move to Level II after 6 straight weeks of clean screens b. After returns to Level I: move to Level II after 4 straight weeks of clean screens	1. Earn 24 points per week 2. Earn MVP[a] 3. Points can buy incentives from the reward menu 4. After 4 weeks of clean screens in Level II, move to Level III	Develop maintenance plan: 1. Negotiate new list of incentives 2. Create new reward menu based on this list 3. If vouchers have been used, they will no longer be applied
Dirty Screen	1. Earn 0 points 2. Lose MVP[a] 3. Cannot cash in points until next clean screen	1. Earn 0 points 2. Immediately return to Level I and stay in Level I until 4 straight weeks of clean screens 3. Lose MVP[a] 4. Cannot cash in points until next clean screen	Therapist, youth, and family determine consequences of dirty screens when maintenance plan is developed

[a]MVP = most valued privilege.

HANDOUT 6.2

List of Potential Rewards Example

Type of reward	What I get	What I want	What caregiver provides
Transportation*	Ride to recreation center once a week	Borrow the car on Saturday	I usually give him rides 3–4 times a week.
Clothing	One outfit at the start of the school year and at Christmas	At least one new outfit a month	I buy him new clothes or shoes once a month or so.
Favorite dessert/snack	Never	Every day	3–4 times per week I usually fix him spaghetti, fried fish, pound cake, and chocolate chip cookies.
Meals	She cooks dinner, sometimes makes breakfast, and packs my lunch	Nothing	I cook every day. I make him breakfast and pack his lunch or give him lunch money.
Laundry	Once a week	Once a week	Once a week I do his laundry, and sometimes I will wash something he wants to wear. I also iron his clothes when he asks.
TV use	Daily	Daily	Daily. I also bought him X-box, which he plays every day. I buy him games once in a while.
Curfew	7:30 P.M. during the week and 9:00 P.M. on weekends	9:00 P.M. during the week and midnight on weekends	I am following probation orders.
Have a friend visit	Every day	Nothing	His friends are always at our house.
Invite friend sleepover	Never	1–2 times per month	I have not allowed this.

(cont.)

Type of reward	What I get	What I want	What caregiver provides
Non-drug/alcohol party/ get-together	Never	At least for my birthday	I have not done this.
Pet/pet supplies	None	A pit bull	We cannot afford.
Privacy time	Never	Wants own room	We cannot afford.
Trips w/family/friends	No	Wants to go to local amusement park	We have not done this.
Car (registration, insurance, payments)	No	Wants a car	We cannot afford.
Phone	A cell phone	Has a cell phone	We gave him a cellphone.
Computer	No	Wants a computer	We cannot afford.
Weights/sports equipment	Some weights	More equipment	He wants a bench/weights.
Music player/iPod	Daily	Have stereo—daily use wants iPod	He uses stereo daily. May get iPod.
Play football	Weekly in fall	Wants to stay on team	He plays; I try and support him.
Other item: jewelry	Ring last fall	Bracelets, rings, necklace	I bought him a ring for his birthday.
Other item:	Report to my probation officer	Good report once a month	I tell the truth—bad reports.

*Most valued privilege.

HANDOUT 6.3

Reward Menu Example

Rewards/Privileges	Cost
Drug Abstinence	
(1) Driving	*MVP When youth has a clean screen, he may borrow car for approved activity on Saturday until 9 P.M.
(2) Clothing	1 point = $1 in therapist vouchers to local store
(3) Party (parent supervised/approved friends, no drugs or alcohol)	30 points
(4) Day trip with parents and one friend	20 points—youth and caregivers to agree on place in future
(5) iPod Shuffle	50 points
(6) New iPod music or CDs	1 point = $1 in music voucher from therapist or parent
(7) Ring/bracelet/jewelry	1 point = $1 from parent toward purchase
(8) Weight-lifting supplies	1 point = $2 from parent toward purchase of supplies
Rewards for Responsible Behavior in Other Domains (optional)	
School Attendance	
(1) Laundry	Full attendance at school that week
(2) Approved friend can spend night	Full attendance at school for 2 weeks
Respectful Behavior	
(1) Making dinner and packing lunch	Respectful to family/others that day

*MVP = most valued privilege.

HANDOUT 6.4

Checkbook Example

Name: Tony

Record all deposits or payments that affect your account.

Date	Description of transaction	Deposit/ Credit (+)		Payment/ Debit (–)		Balance	
1/12	Start treatment	+25	00			25	00
1/12 (week 1)	UDS not clean (cannot spend points)	+0	00			25	00
1/20 (week 2)	UDS clean (1/20) (able to spend points)	+12	.00			37	00
1/22	Check 1 for iTunes music card			–15	00	22	00
2/3 (week 3)	UDS not clean (cannot spend points)	+0	.00			22	00
2/10 (week 4)	Missed appointment, mom called, wants to increase frequency of UDS to 2/week (cannot spend points)					22	00
2/18 (week 5a)	UDS dirty (cannot spend points)	+0.	00			22	00
2/20 (week 5b)	UDS clean—is 2nd screen this week so worth 12 ÷ 2 = 6 points (able to spend points)	+6	.00			28	00
2/21	Check 2 for cell phone minutes			–15	00	13	00

HANDOUT 6.5

Personal Checks Example

Date 1/22

PAY TO THE ORDER OF Ms. Evelyn Smith (mom)

Fifteen POINTS 15.00

FOR iTunes music card Tony Smith

Date 2/21

PAY TO THE ORDER OF Ms. Evelyn Smith (mom)

Fifteen POINTS 15.00

FOR Cell phone minutes Tony Smith

Sample Dialogue: The Point-and-Level Reward System

TASK 6.1: INTRODUCING THE POINT-AND-LEVEL REWARD SYSTEM AND CONTRACT

Therapist: [to Tony and his caregiver] Now that we have gone over the homework assignment, I would like to talk about our tasks for today. We are beginning to understand what things trigger Tony's drug use, and it's time for us to make a plan that will help Tony stay clean. In this treatment, we will do that by:

1. A signed contract, outlining the rewards Tony will get if he is able to stay clean and the privileges he will lose if he does not stay clean.
2. A written reward menu outlining the rewards Tony receives if he stays clean and the privileges removed if he has dirty screens. We call this the *point-and-level system.*

Together, our job is to help Tony get more fun and excitement from staying clean than from using drugs. For example, last week Tony said that one of his main triggers for calling John and ultimately using drugs was boredom—he was bored, so he called John. Boredom is a very common trigger, and our job is to make sure that the rewards we give Tony for being clean will also promote him to do things that are good for him, and will fill up his day and decrease his boredom. Because Tony has been using drugs for awhile, he might have a hard time getting clean at first, and while we want him to not use any drugs at all, if he does use, we will consider it a slip and an opportunity for us to learn what went wrong in the treatment. This will help us make a better plan to help Tony get clean. So, instead of getting upset with him when he uses, I'm going to ask that you to just follow through with the consequences we will set. If we keep following through with the rewards and consequences *every time* we get a drug screen, he should do better over time.

Now, the next step is for us to go over the contract in more detail. Here is a copy of the contract we will use [copies to both Tony and caregiver]. The contract outlines our point-and-level system and describes what Tony will have to do to earn some special privileges that we will set up together after we sign the contract.

The contract has a lot of details in it, and can be a little overwhelming, so it may help to look at this table as we go along (*Point-and-Level System at a Glance* [Handout 6.1]). But once you get used to it, it will make sense, and we know that this type of treatment can work well for youth like Tony. Let's read through the contract together.

[Session continues as the therapist reads entire contract with the family.]

THERAPIST TASK 6.2: COMPLETING A REWARD MENU

Step 1: Explain Concept of Rewards to the Youth and Caregiver

Therapist: [to Tony and his caregiver] Now, we are all going to figure out what Tony's rewards should be if he has clean screens. [Makes the following points.]

- It is very important that we pick things that Tony really likes for rewards as these will have to compete with drug use, so they will need to be something he really wants.
- Many different things can be a reward such as items like CDs and clothes, privileges such as staying up later and using the phone, or activities such as going to the movies.
- Before we can decide on rewards, I need a complete understanding of everything that Tony currently gets as a reward or privilege.
- First, I will meet with Tony and make a list of what privileges and rewards he gets and what rewards he would like to get. Then I will go over the list with Ms. Smith. Once Ms. Smith and I decide on what makes sense for rewards, we will all meet and go over it together. Remember, the caregiver has the final say on all rewards.
- Also, we will need to decide on what Tony's MVP is, the one privilege he cares about the most.

Step 2: Develop List of Potential Rewards with the Youth

Use with *List of Potential Rewards* (Form 6.2) and corresponding *List of Potential Rewards Example* (Handout 6.2).

Therapist: [to Tony] I'm going to mention some things that other teenagers your age often get from their parents. I'd like for you to let me know what you get and what you would like to get for each category. I'll write it down as we go. So let's start with transportation. Do your parents take you places you need to go?

Tony: Yeah, they give me a ride to the rec center sometimes.

Therapist: How often?

Tony: About once a week.

Therapist: What else would you like from your parents regarding transportation?

Tony: I'd like to borrow the car on Saturday nights.

Therapist: Okay, let me write that down, and let's go to the next type of privilege on the list. What kinds of clothes do your parents buy for you?

Tony: I get an outfit when I start school and at Christmas time.

Therapist: What would you like to get?

Tony: Some shoes every couple of months, some clothes every month.

Therapist: How about meals—does your mother or stepdad cook for you?

Tony: Yeah, my parents cook supper most school nights, sometimes they make my breakfast. My mom packs my lunch for school.

Therapist: [Goes through entire list with Tony.] Tony, of all these rewards that we have reviewed, which one do you value the most?

Tony: Driving. I really want to use the car.

Therapist: Okay, I can ask your caregiver to add driving as your MVP to your contract for staying clean. But before we ask, let's make sure this makes sense. Have you ever driven the car before alone and do your parents have insurance for you?

Tony: Yes, they used to let me drive, before they found out about the pot.

Therapist: Now that your parents are probably not going to let you have the car just anytime, is there a certain day of the week and time you may be able to ask for it?

Tony: Saturdays, I could ask to use it on Saturday nights. I'll be home before 10:00 P.M.

Therapist: Okay, we can put that down for now, but we may need to find a backup, so think about your second choice for MVP.

If vouchers/gift certificates are provided by the therapist:

Therapist: Looking over your wish list, which of these things do you think it will make sense to use the vouchers for? Remember, you can get up to 100 dollars worth in coupons from me if your drug screens are clean.

Tony: How about clothes and a CD player?

Therapist: Okay, those sounds reasonable, but remember, your caregiver will have the final decision.

Tony: I know.

Therapist: We reimburse the points at 1 dollar per point. For instance, you would pay me 15 points to get a 15-dollar gift card.

Step 3: Create *Reward Menu* (Form 6.3) with the Caregiver

Use with *List of Potential Rewards* (Form 6.2) and *Reward Menu* (Form 6.3).

Therapist: [to caregiver] Okay, I'm going to review my session with Tony to get your perspective on some things, and then we can decide what privileges make the most sense for him to try and earn. Also, I want to remind you that I am going to help your family find privileges that don't cost money.

Caregiver: Good, because we don't have much money, and I am worried that I might not be able to afford this treatment.

Therapist: I hear what you are saying. As we are going through this process, please speak up and tell me if there are any things I am trying to put into place that don't seem affordable. We don't want to commit your family to privileges you cannot afford.

If vouchers/gift certificates are provided by the therapist:

Therapist: You may remember that our agency can provide up to 100 dollars in gift certificates for Tony to help motivate him to get clean. When I talked to Tony about how he wanted to use these rewards, he said that he would like to use some of the gift certificates in exchange for points to buy clothes or CDs. What do you think about that?

Caregiver: That's fine as long as I get to approve what he buys. I don't like some of that rude music the kids listen to.

Therapist: Of course, I would encourage you to monitor what he buys with the certificates.

Good. Now I'd like to review what Tony told me about privileges he is getting and some things that he would like. I would like for you to do a few things:

1. *Clarify*—tell me what you see yourself and the family as providing.
2. *Comment* on what he wants—let me know which things are realistic or can be given with minor changes and which things are out of the question.
3. *Decide* whether these are rewards you *can give* if clean and *not give* if dirty. I will write your responses as we go.

Oh, another really important point: We want to make sure that we do not put anything on this list that is so *healthy* for Tony that it *should be given anyway* or that may *make him more likely to use drugs.*

Caregiver: Okay, what do you mean by healthy?

Therapist: By healthy, I mean things like going to school, playing sports, or being in a positive after-school activity. The reason we don't want to put these activities on the reward menu is that we don't want to get into a situation in which we are making him earn and pay for things that could actually help him get drug-free. If we keep him home from these activities, he might be more likely to use.

Caregiver: He wants to play basketball. I was thinking I could make him stay clean to play. But it sounds like you are saying I shouldn't do that.

Therapist: Right, it is tempting to try and motivate him with basketball, but that could backfire if he can't get clean at first. Yet we can leverage off his interest in basketball. We could have him earn things like new shoes or sports equipment.

Caregiver: That makes sense. I know he wants some new basketball shoes.

Therapist: Okay, good. Let's keep that in mind.

Therapist: The first thing on the list is transportation. Tony said that you take him to the recreation center about once a week. Does that seem about right? Are there other places you take him?

Caregiver: I do take him to the recreation center about once a week, and I also take him to the store a couple of times a week. I give him rides to John's house sometimes and to school if it's raining.

Therapist: [Goes over each item on Tony's list with his caregiver.] Great, now that we have gone over the whole list, it's time to pick the MVP. This is one of the most important things we will do today. In the near future, we will be getting drug screens on Tony at least once a week. If they are clean, it is going to be very important that Tony be able to receive the MVP, and if they are dirty, he must *not* get this privilege, no matter what.

Therapist: Can you guess what Tony's MVP was?

Caregiver: Driving the car.

Therapist: Yep, he really wants to drive the car. What do you think about this?

Caregiver: I guess that sounds all right. I mean as long as we are sure he is clean.

Therapist: Yes? Well, we will need to be very careful in setting this up. What should the rules be around his use of the car? Think about exactly when he can have it, who he can and cannot be with, where he can go, and how you will check in on him.

Caregiver: Well, I want him home by 9:00 P.M., and I want to know where he is going and who will be with him. I think we are going to have to put John on the list of people who cannot be in the car.

Therapist: I agree, so let's write down that Tony can have the car on Saturday evenings, but he must be home by 9:00 P.M. Also, Tony must tell you where he is going and who will be with him in your car. Tony can give you the names and telephone numbers of each friend who will be with him so that you can call their parents to make sure Tony is giving you accurate information. If Tony is with a friend who you do not approve of, like John, then you can tell him this person is not allowed to be in your car.

Now let's look at the rest of the list again since we had to change it quite a bit. Going down the list, here is what we decided. It makes sense to keep earning desserts, clothing, friends spending the night, iPod, weights, jewelry, laundry, and trips with the family on the list. We've decided to take basketball team membership off the list because you believe it helps him stay out of trouble. I helped you decide to take cell phone off the list because, based on the ABC assessment we completed last week, I'm predicting that we will need to control his cell phone use as it seems to serve as a trigger for meeting with friends who use drugs. Curfew was taken off the list for similar reasons. We determined that it would be too hard for you to not let his friends come over, as they currently do that everyday, and you prefer to have them in your home where you can see them. General TV use was too hard to take away as well, so this was removed. Finally, we decided to eliminate pets, stereo, private room, and owning a car from the list as they are not reasonable goals for your family at this time.

Now it's time to decide which rewards you think should be linked with abstinence and which will work better with other goals on our individualized treatment plan. As you know, we need to keep tracking his school attendance and respectful behavior toward family members. It is important that we have totally separate rewards for each behavior we are trying to help Tony achieve, because if the rewards overlap, it might become confusing or hard to follow the plan. [Decides, with the caregiver, which rewards to link with other problems.]

Let me summarize: We have decided that since school truancy is a big problem, you will tie *school attendance* to one of these rewards that is meaningful for Tony and can be given by you routinely. We will have to check with Tony, but it seems to make sense to place the rewards of *laundry* and *having an approved friend spend the night* on the bottom of our list under the title *school attendance.* You have decided that you will do Tony's laundry for him each weekend if he attends school the week before. You will be calling the school office each Friday to make sure he attended all classes before giving out this reward. When Tony attends school without any absences for 2 weeks in a row, an approved friend may spend the night.

You also decided that you will make *Tony's dinner and pack his lunch for school when he has been respectful to you and other family members that day.* If he is disrespectful, as evidenced by shouting or anger outbursts, he will be required to pack his own lunch for the next school day and to prepare his own dinner, like a sandwich or similar item. So I will create a category called *respectful behavior* and move the rewards of *making dinner and packing lunch* under this heading.

Now it is time to assign points to other rewards that will be used to help Tony get off drugs. We will assign points to all remaining rewards, except the MVP.

Caregiver: Why not assign points to the MVP?

Therapist: We will not need to assign points to Tony's MVP, as he will earn that each week that his screen is clean or lose it if the screen is dirty. We want to make sure that the cost of each reward makes sense given your resources and the number of points Tony can earn each week.

[With the caregiver, goes over the first part of list, assigning cost points to each reward.] Let's look at what we have written down. A top reward on Tony's list is clothing, and we have decided that he may choose to reimburse the gift certificates we provide for clothing or that you will give him a dollar for each point earned. So we will put "1 dollar/point" in the "Cost" column. The next item is having a party with approved friends. This will cost your family an evening's worth of time and about $50 for refreshments. Importantly, Tony is very motivated to have this party, so we've decided that this privilege should cost 50 points. [With the caregiver, completes list, assigning points.]

Great. Now I would like to bring Tony in so that we can go over the list with him to finalize our plans.

Step 4: Confirm and Finalize the *Reward Menu* (Form 6.3) with the Youth and Caregiver

Use with *List of Potential Rewards* (Form 6.2) and *Reward Menu* (Form 6.3).

Therapist: Tony, here is a copy of the *Reward Menu* (Form 6.3). As you can see, you and your mom agree on many of the rewards that your family is currently providing for you. It was a pretty big list, so your mom and I went over it carefully to see what rewards made sense to keep. We tried to make sure that the list included things that were important to you, would not put you at risk to use drugs, and could be provided by your parents. We also assigned a cost to each reward. Let's look at the list together, and I will explain more about the decisions we made if you have questions.

As you predicted, we took a pet pit bull off the list for now, but there are a number of things here that you asked for. Importantly, your mom agreed that driving should be added as your MVP for staying clean. She really liked your idea of earning the car once a week for not using drugs. Let's add driving as the MVP on the *Reward Menu* (Form 6.3). You have to make sure you are home by 9:00 P.M., and you need to give your mom the names and telephone numbers of all friends who will be with you. John is not allowed to ride in the car. Also, you need to tell your parents where you will be taking the car as well. Keep in mind that your parents have to approve where you are going and who will be with you, all right?

Tony: Okay. Driving is the most important thing to me.

[Therapist then reviews all of the other rewards from the reward menu with Tony and his caregiver to finalize the contract and solicit any questions and/or feedback.]

TASK 6.3: MONITORING POINTS EARNED AND EXCHANGED WITH THE CHECKBOOK SYSTEM

Therapist: I need to introduce you to one other aspect of the point-and-level system. I would like to talk to you about how to best track the points that Tony earns and spends as he goes through treatment. We use a tracking system that is modeled after checkbooks used by the bank. Teens Tony's age tend to like this system, and it can help teach Tony money-handling skills.

Tony: I know how to handle money.

Caregiver: Yeah, my money.

Therapist: So Tony, it sounds like this method will be perfect for you.

Tony: What do I have to do?

Therapist: Let's look at these forms. Here are the types of checks we will use and the sheet we will use to keep our records. [Passes out *Checkbook* (Form 6.4) and *Personal Checks* (Form 6.5).] These are the same types of checks and records adults use when they track the spending in their bank accounts.

Caregiver: So he will write me or you a check when he wants to cash in points he has earned?

Therapist: Correct, and we (you or I) will go to the *Checkbook* (Form 6.4) balance sheet and make sure Tony has the necessary points before we cash his check.

Tony: How does the balance sheet work?

Therapist: Here, let's look at an example that will make it easier to explain. [Passes out *Checkbook Example* (Handout 6.4) and *Personal Checks Example* (Handout 6.5).] Let's fill the forms out for you. I will write this on mine, and Tony, you fill in your *Checkbook* (Form 6.4) as well. We need two copies, one for my chart and one for you and your family. Start by putting in today's date and 25 points in the credit column. That will give you a balance of 25 points today.

Tony: So I write that in?

Caregiver: Right, put a 25 in the balance. You have 25 points starting today.

Tony: Cool, can I write a check?

Therapist: You know better than that. Remember the rules we made when we signed the contract? Let's go over them again. [Reviews the following points from the contract.]

- You will keep track of your points with a checkbook and write checks to your caregiver or therapist to cash in points.
- You may only spend points when your most recent drug screen and breath scan are clean.
- You may only spend points that you have already earned; in other words, you cannot go into debt in your checkbook or spend points you have not yet earned.
- You may have access to your MVP, driving, when your most recent screen and scan are clean.
- You may not have access to your MVP, driving, when the most recent screen and scan are dirty.
- If you ever skip or avoid a screen, it will be considered dirty, and your MVP will be taken away.

- You will earn 12 points per week in Level I for clean screens and scans.
- When you have been clean for 6 weeks in a row, you will advance to Level II.
- In Level II, you will earn a total of 24 points (12 bonus points) for each week your screens are clean.
- Just like in Level I, in Level II you will continue to earn your MVP and be able to write checks to spend points for rewards when your screens and scans are clean.
- If you have more than one screen a week, the point value of each screen will be 12 (in Level I) or 24 (in Level II) divided by the number of screens. So, for example, if you get two screens a week in Level I, each will be worth 6 points.

Tony: Okay, so I have to give a urine screen to be able to spend my 25 points?

Therapist: Right, and it has to be clean. You can only get your MVP and spend points when you are clean.

Tony: So what if it takes me a month to get clean?

Caregiver: No car for a month. You keep your points, but you cannot cash them in.

Therapist: Right, and you may not have any privilege on the list here—until you are clean and can buy it.

Tony: Okay, you guys have made your point. When do I get screened?

Therapist: Well, we are out of time today, but drug screening just happens to be the next topic we will cover. We will probably be getting a drug screen from you during our session next week.

Tony: Guess I better work hard on my plans this week.

Therapist: Yes, please try to follow the self-management plans we discussed last week. I hope you will be able to test clean next week. That would be a great way to start.

Caregiver: Maybe we should review those plans for a minute.

Therapist: Good idea.

[Therapist and family review self-management plans in place for triggers the youth is likely to encounter before the next session.]

CHAPTER 7

Drug Testing Protocol

THERAPIST GOAL

1. **Provide caregivers with a reliable and valid measure of substance use so that contingencies can be applied appropriately and quickly.**

This chapter describes the drug testing protocol that is discussed and established after the therapist and caregiver have agreed on the specifics of the CM point-and-level system. This protocol can be used to monitor drug use as long as that drug can be reliably and routinely detected by available urine screens or breath scans.

OVERVIEW OF DRUG TESTING PROTOCOL

Helping caregivers develop the skills to obtain urine drug screens and breath tests is an important part of treatment, because caregivers are best positioned to obtain these screens. This process also empowers caregivers to monitor their youth more carefully and can help the family generalize gains after treatment ends. Most caregivers are able to learn how to conduct screens on their own after first observing the therapist go through the protocol, then walking through the steps as they are outlined on the *Caregiver Handout for Conducting Drug Screens* (Handout 7.1). As noted previously, behavioral contingencies are most effective when administered consistently, precisely, and on the basis of objective evidence (Budney & Higgins, 1998). Random urine drug screens and alcohol breath scans are the preferred methods used to provide this objective evidence.

Why Objective Measures of Drug Use Should Be Obtained

There are three very important reasons for using objective measures.

1. Even with the best of intentions to stop using illicit drugs, adolescents who abuse drugs often do not tell the truth about their substance use. Consequently, an adolescent's verbal report, while seemingly genuine and heartfelt, might not accurately reflect current drug use.
2. Because the purpose of CM is to increase incentives for abstinence, providing rewards without adequate verification (objective evidence) will undermine the program's integrity and, more important, will be insufficient to compete with existing drug use contingencies.
3. Objective monitoring coupled with negative (i.e., clean) results will set the stage for the youth to begin rebuilding trust with his or her caregivers. A positive parent–adolescent affective bond (e.g., what my parents think about me) is often reported as a main reason that keeps youth from using drugs.

Introducing Drug Testing

The drug testing protocol can be reviewed with the caregiver and youth at any point in the process of introducing CM that seems clinically appropriate. The review of this protocol should include a brief rationale for drug testing, a description of the frequency of testing, and a discussion of what should happen if the youth either refuses to or cannot provide a specimen. It is important to highlight for the caregivers that the youth should *not* know when testing will occur. Some therapists prefer to start CM with urine drug screen collection, because such testing is a central component of the intervention and can provide concrete evidence of the problem that needs to be addressed. Others prefer to wait until the other CM components have been introduced. An important clinical caveat is that youth should not receive multiple urine drug screens that are not tied to rewards or consequences. Hence, it is recommended that drug screening and breath scans not occur on a routine basis until the *Point-and-Level System Contract for Youth and Caregiver* (Form 6.1) has been signed and a *Reward Menu* (Form 6.3) put into place to structure the rewards and consequences tied to the results.

Guidelines for Collecting Urine Specimens

The main goal of this procedure is to ensure that an unaltered urine specimen is obtained. As such, step-by-step guidelines for urine collection are provided by the *Urine Drug Testing Instructions for Therapists* (Information Sheet 7.1) and *Caregiver Handout for Conducting Drug Screens* (Handout 7.1). These guidelines, however, might need to be modified depending on the organization or site where the therapist is employed to ensure compliance with agency standards. The following information is derived from the U.S. Department of Health and Human Services Mandatory Guidelines for Federal

Workplace Drug Testing Programs. A copy of this guideline can be found at *workplace.samhsa.gov.*

Where to Collect Specimens

The collection site will most likely be the youth's home or the agency outpatient clinic. Before using a site, the monitoring adult should check for the presence of adulterants or containers of urine that might have been placed there by the youth. The adult should remove all cleaning solutions and potential adulterants from the bathroom prior to collection.

Position of the Observer

These suggestions should only be followed if consistent with agency procedures and guidelines. *When a same-gender caregiver is available,* the caregiver should be positioned (i.e., stand) in the doorway of the bathroom where any suspicious activity can be observed, but without directly viewing the youth's genitalia. When a *different-gender caregiver or the therapist is available,* steps need to be taken to ensure visual privacy, but the caregiver or therapist should be positioned near enough to hear any attempts the youth might make to alter the specimen. Thus, it might make sense to leave the door open and have the caregiver or therapist stand outside the door, around the corner, or facing away from the youth.

Adulterants

Products to mask the presence of drugs in urine are readily available on the market and are constantly being produced and modified. To find out more about these agents, consult the National Institute on Drug Abuse website (*www.nida.nih.gov*), or call a local laboratory. Carefully following the procedures on *Urine Drug Testing Instructions for Therapists* (Information Sheet 7.1) and *Caregiver Handout for Conducting Drug Screens* (Handout 7.1) will help minimize risk of adulterants.

Guidelines for Collecting Alcohol Breath Specimens

The main goal of this procedure is to assist families in detecting youth alcohol use when such use is posing a potential clinical problem. Step-by-step guidelines for breath scan collection are provided on the *Caregiver Handout for Collecting Alcohol Breath Specimens* (Handout 7.3) instruction page.

When to Collect Specimens

Because alcohol breath scans have a narrow detection window (several minutes to hours after last use, depending on amount of use and how rapidly the youth metabolizes alcohol), families should collect the breath scans at times when the youth is either at high risk for recent use (e.g., returning home from being out with peers) or shows signs or symptoms of intoxication (e.g., red eyes, unsteady gait, unusual affect or behavior). On the basis of the youth's history and symptoms, therapists should work with the youth and caregiver to determine whether breath scans are indicated and, if so, how often they will be administered, by whom, and under what circumstances. As a general rule of thumb, youth who are known to abuse alcohol should have routine breath scans written into their contract and should be tested at high-risk times at least two to three times a week. Youth who have another primary drug of abuse but use alcohol intermittently should also be expected to give breath scans at times when they might be at increased risk or demonstrating symptoms of alcohol and drug use. Note that information provided in the ABC assessment might be helpful in determining high-risk times. Therapists and caregivers can also choose to administer breath scans each time a urine screen is collected. They should be aware, however, that unless the youth has had the opportunity to use alcohol within an hour or so of the screen collection, results will likely be negative regardless of the youth's recent history of alcohol use.

How to Collect Specimens

The procedures for collecting alcohol breath scans are described step by step in the *Caregiver Handout for Collecting Alcohol Breath Specimens* (Handout 7.3). In summary, caregivers unwrap the tube, squeeze the middle to break the inner glass ampoule, and then have the youth take a deep breath and exhale in one continuous motion for 12 seconds into the end of the tube designated by an arrow. Caregivers then shake the tube to distribute the crystals evenly and wait 2 minutes before trying to identify a change in the crystal's colors. For clean tests, the tube crystals will not change color. For positive (dirty) tests, the crystals will develop a gray to blue/green cast.

Aims and Time Frame of the Following Tasks

The primary goal of the following tasks is to help caregivers learn how to collect urine drug screens and alcohol breath tests so that the youth can be carefully and consistently monitored for substance use and appropriate contingencies can be applied. A secondary goal is to empower caregivers to generalize their skills so that they can provide better monitoring of potential substance use after treatment ends. Often therapists are able to introduce the concept and rules for drug testing in about 15 minutes. It might take an additional 15 to 20 minutes to gather the specimens from the youth and read test results.

THERAPIST TASK 7.1: INTRODUCING DRUG TESTING

Objective

1. Provide general information about the timing and process of conducting urine drug screens and alcohol breath scans.

Material

- *Therapist Checklist 7.1: Introducing the Drug Testing Protocol*

Accomplishing the Objective

Following the steps outlined in *Therapist Checklist 7.1: Introducing the Drug Testing Protocol*, the therapist describes the important role that objective substance use screening plays in CM, the timing of drug screens and alcohol breath scans, and the location of testing. The therapist then schedules a time, unbeknownst to the youth, when the caregiver will administer the first substance testing.

THERAPIST TASK 7.2: GUIDELINES FOR COLLECTING URINE SPECIMENS

Objectives

1. Conduct a drug screen with the youth to demonstrate procedures to caregivers.
2. Teach caregivers to obtain an unaltered urine specimen.
3. Teach caregivers to interpret the results of the urine drug test.
4. Answer youth or caregiver questions about reliability and validity of drug testing.

Materials

- *Therapist Checklist 7.2: Teaching Caregivers to Conduct Urine Drug Screens*
- *Caregiver Handout for Conducting Drug Screens* (Handout 7.1)
- *Drug and Alcohol Testing Resource List* (Handout 7.2)
- *Urine Drug Testing Instructions for Therapists* (Information Sheet 7.1)
- *Frequently Asked Questions about the Integrated E-Z Split Key Three-Panel Cup* (Information Sheet 7.2)
- *Frequently Asked Questions about the Integrated E-Z Split Key Six-Panel Cup* (Information Sheet 7.3)

Accomplishing the Objectives

The purpose of this task is to teach the caregivers reliable and valid procedures for collecting urine specimens from their adolescent for drug testing. This task is accomplished by modeling and instruction. The therapist should first give a copy of the *Caregiver Handout for Conducting Drug Screens* (Handout 7.1) to the caregivers. This handout provides a detailed and simple protocol for collecting the urine specimen, including the necessary preparation for collection, procedures to follow when collecting the specimen, how to read the results, and how to discard the testing materials. The therapist should briefly review these procedures with the youth and caregivers.

Next, the therapist demonstrates how the urine specimen should be collected, using the adolescent as an example. *Urine Drug Testing Instructions for Therapists* (Information Sheet 7.1) gives a step-by-step procedure that the therapist can model for the caregivers, checking off each step as it is completed. After the specimen is collected, the therapist helps the youth and caregiver read the results, per instructions given in Handout 7.1 and Information Sheet 7.1. Returning to the *Caregiver Handout for Conducting Drug Screens* (Handout 7.1), the therapist should review the procedures with the caregivers one more time to confirm that they are understood.

Finally, the therapist answers any questions the family members might have, such as whether the youth can test positive for marijuana from secondhand smoke and whether any legal medications can trigger positive results. *Frequently Asked Questions about the Integrated E-Z Split Key Three-Panel Cup* (Information Sheet 7.2) and *Six-Panel Cup* (Information Sheet 7.3) provide answers to some common client questions. In addition, the *Drug and Alcohol Testing Resource List* (Handout 7.2) is provided to assist the therapist or caregiver in accessing other validated drug and alcohol testing kits.

THERAPIST TASK 7.3: GUIDELINES FOR COLLECTING ALCOHOL BREATH SPECIMENS (AS NEEDED)

Objectives

1. Obtain an appropriate breath specimen.
2. Teach caregivers to obtain a breath specimen.
3. Teach caregivers to interpret the results of the breath scan.

Materials

- *Therapist Checklist 7.3: Collecting Alcohol Breath Specimens*
- *Caregiver Handout for Collecting Alcohol Breath Specimens* (Handout 7.3)

Accomplishing the Objectives

As noted previously, breath specimens are collected when alcohol use is suspected and, because of the narrow detection window, at times when recent use is most likely (e.g., after visiting friends on a weekend night). Collecting breath specimens is much easier than collecting urine screens, and the therapist demonstrates the procedure and has the caregivers conduct a test during the session. *Caregiver Handout for Collecting Alcohol Breath Specimens* (Handout 7.3) provides step-by-step instructions for collecting and interpreting breath scans for both therapists and caregivers, and the therapist should give the caregiver and youth a copy. The steps described in this handout should be briefly reviewed and then demonstrated by the therapist, carefully interpreting the results. The practitioner should then guide the caregivers through the same testing process.

TROUBLESHOOTING TIPS

Objective

The purpose of this section is to help therapists anticipate common challenges to urine drug screen and breath scan collection and to suggest strategies to address these difficulties.

Challenges and Solutions

The Caregiver Is Uncomfortable or Refuses to Collect the Specimen.

The therapist should identify the caregiver's concerns and attempt to address them. The therapist might agree to collect specimens at the office until the caregiver feels more comfortable or until his or her concerns are addressed. Often showing caregivers what to do and walking them through the process several times helps alleviate their concerns. Alternatively, the therapist and caregiver might identify someone else in the family network who can collect the specimens (with appropriate consent).

There Are Privacy Concerns Related to Gender or Family History.

At times, the therapist might feel that it is clinically contraindicated for some caregivers to visually monitor the youth's urine drug screen collection. In these cases, the therapist can have caregivers follow the *Caregiver Handout for Conducting Drug Screens* (Handout 7.1) protocol carefully as visual observation is not required. The therapist might also want to have caregivers obtain assistance from another, more appropriate family member or social support to help with this task.

The Youth Refuses to Provide a Screen or Breath Scan.

Arguments with the youth should be avoided. However, the youth should be reminded of the consequence for not providing a specimen (i.e., counts as dirty screen). If the youth fails to comply within 30 minutes, the consequence should be enforced.

The Youth Has Difficulty Urinating.

Having the youth drink a glass of water or running warm water over his or her hands in the sink can help produce a urine specimen.

The Youth Uses Alcohol as Well as Marijuana.

If alcohol use or abuse is suspected, the therapist should also screen for this substance. Such screening can most easily be accomplished with disposable alcohol breath detection scans. As noted previously, several products are available on the market (see *Drug and Alcohol Testing Resource List* [Handout 7.2]). The *Caregiver Handout for Collecting Alcohol Breath Specimens* (Handout 7.3) provides instructions for obtaining and reading alcohol breath scans. The therapist should incorporate at least one weekly random alcohol breath test, conducted by the caregiver immediately after a high-risk time, into the CM contract. All rewards should then be contingent on having *both* clean drug *and* clean alcohol screens each week.

The Youth Uses Other Drugs as Well as Marijuana.

CM can be used to treat a drug of abuse as long as that drug can be reliably and routinely detected by urine screens, breath scans, or other scientifically proven methods. Routine affordable urine screening tests can be purchased that test for a number of drugs such as marijuana, cocaine, amphetamines, opiates, benzodiazepines, or methamphetamines (i.e., ecstasy or crystal meth). See the *Drug and Alcohol Testing Resource List* (Handout 7.2) for more information on how to access some of the numerous drug testing kits currently available on the market.

The therapist who suspects other drug use in addition to marijuana should consider obtaining a urine screen for all suspected substances at intake and repeat this screen every 3 to 4 weeks throughout treatment. If the youth is being treated for the use of drugs that have a shorter detection window than marijuana, he or she will need to be tested more frequently. The following table provides a quick reference of the average time that drug metabolites can be found in urine specimens. If the youth tests positive for another drug or shows signs or symptoms of other drug use, the frequency of drug screens should be increased based on the detection times for this drug until the youth has tested clean for a reasonable period of time.

Average Detection Times for Abused Substances

Drug	Urine detection time
Amphetamines	2–4 days
Barbiturates	2–4 days (phenobarbital, 2 weeks or longer)
Benzodiazepines	Varies—depends on half-life of drug
Cannabinoids (marijuana)	Infrequent user: varies up to 10 days—depends on amount/frequency; chronic users: 30 days or longer
Cocaine metabolite	1–3 days
Methaqualone	Up to 14 days
Opiates	1–3 days
Phencyclidine	2–7 days
Alcohol	Several hours

Note. Based on American Association for Clinical Chemistry (1988).

The Youth Adamantly Denies Using but the Test Result Is Positive.

It is fairly common for youth to deny drug use even in the face of dirty screens, especially early in the treatment process. Several approaches to dealing with a potentially false-positive screen are listed next in the order in which they should be tried.

Clinical Strategies for Managing Potentially False-Positive Screens

- In general, the best initial approach is to continue to follow the rules and contract as outlined, treating the screen as a true-positive (i.e., dirty) result. The therapist might let the youth know, in a nonblaming way, that although results might not be 100% certain, rewards cannot be provided unless positive proof that the youth has not used is obtained. The only way to know this is to gather a clean screen.
- If the youth continues to have screens that might be false positives, the next step is to take the urine to a lab where a more careful *quantitative* screen of the urine can be conducted to obtain drug levels. If these results contradict prior results (i.e., clean at lab), the therapist and caregiver can then choose to reward the youth. The therapist should also consult with the laboratory concerning possible contaminants that might have cross-reacted with the test to produce a false-positive screen.
- Two therapist information sheets are provided that outline common questions concerning two specific drug screens. The first, *Frequently Asked Questions about the Integrated E-Z Split Key Three-Panel Cup* (Information Sheet 7.2), describes a cup that tests for marijuana, cocaine, and amphetamines. The second, *Frequently Asked Questions about the Integrated E-Z Split Key Six-Panel Cup* (Information Sheet 7.3), provides information concerning a cup that tests for methamphetamines, benzodiazepines, and opiates as well as marijuana, cocaine, and amphetamines. If the therapist is using another type of drug detection cup, he or she should obtain information from the manufacturer on that specific test because it might differ from the E-Z Split Key Cups described in the handouts.

The Drug Test Results Yield Faint Lines.

The therapist should follow the recommendations of the drug cup manufacturers concerning faint lines. Recommendations for the Integrated E-Z Split Key Cups described here are to read faint lines as true lines. That is, if a line is partially present, it should be read as fully present.

The Therapist or Caregiver Is Suspicious of Clean Drug Screen Results.

If the therapist or caregiver doubts the outcomes of a urine drug screen, she or he can do one of the following: collect urine from the youth's first morning void, when the urine will be most concentrated; secretly arrange to change the date and timing of the next urine collection so that the youth will not be able to prepare for the test; or send a sample to a lab for confirmation.

The Youth Uses Marijuana Laced with Cocaine.

Because youth may unknowingly use marijuana that has been laced with cocaine, a drug screen may test positive for both drugs. Although it might be difficult to determine whether the youth is using both substances individually or whether the positive cocaine results are a byproduct of his or her marijuana use, frequent retests should help resolve this concern, because cocaine stays in the system for shorter periods of time than marijuana.

THERAPIST CHECKLISTS, HANDOUTS, AND INFORMATION SHEETS FOR CHAPTER 7: DRUG TESTING PROTOCOL

THERAPIST CHECKLIST 7.1

Introducing the Drug Testing Protocol

Case number: ______________ **Session date:** ______________

I have explained that (check each item covered during session):

___ Urine drug screens are a necessary part of CM interventions.

___ Alcohol breath scans can also be part of CM interventions.

___ Urine drug screens and alcohol breath scans will help us know whether (*youth's name*) is using drugs or alcohol and whether treatment is working.

___ Drug screens will be conducted at least one time per week and at random times.

___ Alcohol breath scans will be conducted at times that (*youth's name*) is considered to be at high risk for recent alcohol use.

___ After 10 weeks *in a row* of clean test results, the urine drug screens and alcohol breath scans may decrease in frequency.

___ These urine drug screens and alcohol breath scans may be conducted during treatment sessions, at home, or during unannounced office visits.

___ (*Youth's name*) should be tested at high-risk times (e.g., Saturday night).

___ If (*youth's name*) refuses a urine screen or breath scan, avoids being transported to the office for a screen, or is unable to provide urine within 30 minutes, the screen or scan will be considered dirty.

I have:

___ Scheduled the next urine test and breath scan with caregiver at a time unknown to the youth. [Note: Youth often receive their first test during the current session.]

___ Informed the caregiver that the youth should not be told the date the next testing is scheduled to occur.

___ Asked the youth and caregiver to describe their understanding of the drug testing and breath scan procedures.

___ Asked the youth and caregiver to describe any concerns or questions about the drug testing or breath scan procedures.

THERAPIST CHECKLIST 7.2

Teaching Caregivers to Conduct Urine Drug Screens

Case number: ______________ **Session date:** ______________

I have (check each item covered during session):

___ Provided the youth and caregiver with a copy of the *Caregiver Handout for Conducting Drug Screens* (Handout 7.1).

___ Following the items on *Urine Drug Testing Instructions for Therapists* (Information Sheet 7.1), performed a drug screen with the caregiver and youth to demonstrate the procedure.

___ Explained how to read the results of the drug screen to the caregiver and youth, as described on the *Caregiver Handout for Conducting Drug Screens* (Handout 7.1) and *Urine Drug Testing Instructions for Therapists* (Information Sheet 7.1).

___ Answered any questions or concerns indicated by the youth or caregiver for the aforementioned drug testing protocols and *Frequently Asked Questions about the Integrated E-Z Split Key Three-Panel Cup* (Information Sheet 7.2) and *Six-Panel Cup* (Information Sheet 7.3).

___ Determined the availability of the aforementioned drug screen kits and identified viable alternatives from the *Drug and Alcohol Testing Resource List* (Handout 7.2) if they are not available.

THERAPIST CHECKLIST 7.3

Collecting Alcohol Breath Specimens

Case number: ______________ **Session date:** ______________

I have (check each item covered during session):

___ Provided the youth and caregiver a copy of *Caregiver Handout for Collecting Alcohol Breath Specimens* (Handout 7.3) for conducting breath scans.

___ Performed a breath scan with the caregiver and youth to demonstrate the procedure.

___ Explained how to read the results of the scan to the caregiver and youth.

___ Guided the caregivers in performing a breath scan with the youth.

___ Answered any questions or concerns indicated by the youth or caregiver.

HANDOUT 7.1

Caregiver Handout for Conducting Drug Screens

Note: The following instructions are for a certain kind of cup called Integrated E-Z Split Key Cups. The cups used by your therapist might be different. An asterisk(*) is used to mark steps that might need to be modified. Your therapist will tell you which steps need to be changed and how to do so.

I. Before Collecting the Sample

1. Take everything out of the bathroom that the youth could potentially use to alter the urine specimen (e.g., cleaning solutions, any containers with water, medications).
2. Seal the water faucets with masking tape or a similar adhesive so that they cannot be turned on without breaking the tape.
3. Write the youth's name and the date on the cup.
4. Ask the youth to remove jacket or bulky clothes that might conceal objects.
5. Check the youth's pockets and clothing for anything that could be used to change the test.
6. Put on disposable gloves.
7. Have your watch ready, so that you can time 5 minutes once the test is started.

II. Obtaining the Urine Specimen

1. Ask the youth to provide the specimen (i.e., pee into the cup) with appropriate supervision (stand at the door way facing out—close enough to be able to hear any suspicious activity).
2. When the youth has provided the specimen, have him or her replace the cap on the cup.
3. Take the cup from the youth and place it on a flat surface, making sure the cap is on tight.
4. *Read the temperature strip on the cup and ensure that the urine is between 90 and 100 degrees. (*Remember*: If the urine is not in this temperature range, the youth might have altered the sample—ask for another sample or count as dirty).
5. *Place the cup so that you can view the flat side.
6. *Remove the label covering the test indicators from the flat side of the cup.
7. *Insert the round wheel-like key into the round hole on the side of the cup (you *should hear a click or small noise when the key is inserted correctly*). You do not need to turn the key. Start timing with your watch once the key has been inserted.
8. *After the key is inserted, you will see the urine being absorbed by the testing material.
9. *Read the results 5 minutes after inserting the key.

(cont.)

III. *Reading the Results

Pictures at the top of the flat side of the cup will help you read the results.

1. Two lines indicate that the urine was negative for the drug being tested (clean—no drug detected).
2. One line at the top—by the "C"—indicates that the urine was positive (dirty for the drug being tested).
3. No lines or only one line at the bottom—by the "T"—indicates that the test was not valid and should be repeated.

If unsure of results, call the therapist for help.

Drug name abbreviations on E-Z Split Key Three-Panel Cup:

COC = cocaine

AMP = amphetamine

THC = marijuana

IV. Discarding All Testing Materials

1. Discard urine in toilet.
2. Test cup, tape, and gloves should be disposed of in the trash.

HANDOUT 7.2

Drug and Alcohol Testing Resource List

General Resource

www.nida.nih.gov

Supplies

The following companies sell integrated instant test cups and alcohol breath scans:

UriTox Medical (*www.uritoxmedicaltesting.com*)
3060 W. Sylvania Ave, Suite B
Toledo, OH 43623
(419) 475-2885—phone
(877) 487-4869—phone
(419) 475-2886—fax

BTNX (*www.btnx.com*)
(905) 944-9565—phone
(888) 339-9964—phone
(905) 944-0406—fax

Florida Drug Screening, Inc. (*www.floridadrugscreening.com*)
780 S. Apollo Blvd
Melbourne, FL 32901
(321) 728-2941—phone
(888) 441-4599—phone
(321) 953-6545—fax

Varian, Inc. (*www.varianinc.com*)
(650) 424-5020—phone

DTS—Drug Test Systems (*www.drugtestsystems.com*)
(888) 805-4849—phone

HANDOUT 7.3

Caregiver Handout for Collecting Alcohol Breath Specimens

Note: The following instructions are based on a specific test called BreathScan manufactured by Akers Biosciences, Inc. Instructions may vary depending on the type of breath scan used. An asterisk(*) denotes steps that might differ. Therapists and caregivers should follow the instructions for the specific alcohol breath detection scan they are using if they are different.

I. **Collecting the Sample**

1. Make sure that the breath scan tube is not bent or crushed.
2. Squeeze the middle of the outer plastic tube between your thumb and forefinger to break the inner glass ampoule containing yellow crystals. Use immediately. *Note: Squeeze only once. Do not crush or bend tube.*
3. *Ask the youth to take a deep breath and exhale in one continuous breath for 12 seconds through the end of the tube designated by an arrow. *Note: Have the youth blow very hard. Make sure the youth exhales rather than inhales.*
4. *Shake tester to distribute crystals evenly.
5. *Wait 2 minutes.

II. **Interpreting the Results**

1. *Identify color change of majority of crystals.
   - ***Negative***—no color change in the crystals.
   - ***Positive***—crystals will develop an aqua (blue/green) cast; for best results compare with an unused tester.

INFORMATION SHEET 7.1

Urine Drug Testing Instructions for Therapists

Note: Instructions may vary depending on the type of urine drug screens used. The following instructions are for the Integrated E-Z Split Key Cups. An asterisk(*) is used to denote steps that might differ. Therapists should defer to the instructions specific to the test they are using as indicated.

1. Take everything out of the bathroom that the youth could potentially use to alter the urine specimen (e.g., cleaning solutions).
2. Seal the water faucets with tape so that they cannot be turned on without breaking the tape.
3. Ask the youth to remove jacket or bulky clothes that can conceal objects.
4. Check the youth's pockets and clothing for concealed adulterants.
5. Put on disposable gloves.
6. Take the urine cup from the bag.
7. Write the youth's name and the date on the cup.
8. Remove the top of the cup.
9. Ask the youth to provide the specimen with appropriate supervision (leave the door open wide enough to be able to hear activity in the bathroom).
10. When the youth has provided the specimen, have him or her replace the cap on the cup.
11. *Take the specimen from the youth and place it on a flat surface, making sure the cap is on tight.
12. *Read the temperature strip on the cup and ensure that the urine is between 90 and 100 degrees. If the urine is not in this temperature range, the youth might have altered the sample (ask for another sample or count as dirty).
13. *Place the cup so that you can view the flat side.
14. *Remove the label covering the test indicators from the side of the cup.
15. *Insert the round wheel-like key into the round hole on the side of the cup. You will need to push on the key, and you *should hear a click or small noise when the key is inserted correctly.* You do not need to turn the key.
16. *After the key is inserted, you will see the urine being absorbed by the testing material.
17. *Read the results 5 minutes after inserting the key.
    Pictures at the top of the flat side of the cup will help you read the results. See package insert for a picture demonstrating how to read results.
    - Two lines indicate that the urine was negative for the drug being tested (no drug detected).
    - One line at the top—by the "C"—indicates that the urine was positive (dirty) for the drug being tested (e.g., marijuana).
    - No lines or only one line at the bottom—by the "T"—indicates that the test was not valid. In other words, the cup did not work and the test should be repeated.
18. Discard all testing materials, tape, and gloves.

INFORMATION SHEET 7.2

Frequently Asked Questions about the Integrated E-Z Split Key Three-Panel Cup

1. **What is the shelf-life of the test cups?**

   The test cups have a shelf-life of 18 months from the date of manufacture. The expiration date is indicated on each individual foil pouch, and the cup can be used up until that date.

2. **What are the screening cutoff concentrations?**

   The screening cutoff concentrations of the tests are:

   Amphetamines .... 1,000 ng/ml
   Cannabis .... 50 ng/ml
   Cocaine .... 300 ng/ml

3. **How accurate are the drug tests?**

   Laboratory test results for drugs of abuse have indicated greater than 97% accuracy when used according to the instructions.

4. **Is it possible to test positive for THC (marijuana) from exposure to secondhand smoke?**

   Absolutely not! Urine concentrations of THC above the cutoff sensitivity level of the test, or a positive result, are not possible by exposure to secondhand smoke.

5. **Will commonly used substances such as vitamins, penicillin, aspirin, caffeine, and acetaminophen (Tylenol) affect the results?**

   No. The tests are drug and drug metabolite specific. These commonly taken substances are chemically and structurally different after being metabolized by the body from the drugs being tested for and, therefore, under most circumstances will not interfere with or compromise test results.

6. **Are there any legal medications that can trigger positive results?**

   Yes. Some forms of the drugs tested for may be available legally under prescription as well.

7. **Can stimulants that are taken for attention-deficit disorder/attention-deficit/hyperactivity disorder (ADD/ADHD) affect the results?**

   Yes. Some medications test positive on the amphetamine test (see below).

Potential False-Positive Indicators

Test drug	Some drugs that can cause false-positive preliminary urine tests
Amphetamines	Ephedrine, phenylephrine, amphetamines, dextroamphetamine sulfate (Adderall and Adderall XR), methamphetamine, selegiline, bupropion, desipramine, amantadine
Cocaine	Topical anesthetics containing cocaine
Marijuana	Dronabinol, hemp seed oil

INFORMATION SHEET 7.3

Frequently Asked Questions about the Integrated E-Z Split Key Six-Panel Cup

1. **What is the shelf-life of the test cups?**

   The test cups have a shelf-life of 18 months from the date of manufacture. The expiration date is indicated on each individual foil pouch and can be used up until that date.

2. **What are the screening cutoff concentrations?**

   The screening cutoff concentrations of the tests are as follows:

Drug	Cutoff
Amphetamines	1,000 ng/ml
Benzodiazepines	300 ng/ml
Cannabis	50 ng/ml
Cocaine	300 ng/ml
Methamphetamines	1,000 ng/ml
Opiates	2,000 ng/ml

3. **How accurate are the drug tests?**

   Laboratory test results for drugs of abuse have indicated greater than 97% accuracy when used according to the instructions.

4. **Is it possible to test positive for THC (marijuana) from exposure to secondhand smoke?**

   Absolutely not! Urine concentrations of THC above the cutoff sensitivity level of the test, or a positive result, are not possible by exposure to secondhand smoke.

5. **Will commonly used substances such as vitamins, penicillin, aspirin, caffeine, and acetaminophen (Tylenol) affect the results?**

   No. The tests are drug and drug metabolite specific. These commonly taken substances are chemically and structurally different after being metabolized by the body from the drugs being tested for and, therefore, under most circumstances will not interfere with or compromise test results.

6. **Are there any legal medications that can trigger positive results?**

   Yes. Some forms of the drugs tested for may be available legally under prescription as well.

7. **Can stimulants that are taken for attention-deficit disorder/attention-deficit/hyperactivity disorder (ADD/ADHD) affect the results?**

   Yes. Some medications test positive on both the methamphetamine and amphetamine tests.

(cont.)

8. Will the amphetamine test on the three-panel cup catch methamphetamine (ecstasy) use?

Methamphetamines are metabolized to amphetamines. Therefore, the amphetamine test on the three-panel cup should detect the metabolites of methamphetamine. If the youth's primary drug of abuse is methamphetamine, the six-panel cup should be used periodically for testing because this is a more specific test of methamphetamine and should not cross-react with the stimulant prescription drugs, while the amphetamine test does cross-react with these drugs.

Potential False-Positive Indicators

Test drug	**Some drugs that can cause false-positive preliminary urine tests**
Amphetamines	Ephedrine, phenylephrine, amphetamines, dextroamphetamine sulfate (Adderall and Adderall XR), methamphetamine, selegiline, bupropion, desipramine, amantadine
Cocaine	Topical anesthetics containing cocaine
Marijuana	Dronabinol, hemp seed oil
Methamphetamine	Ranitidine (Pylorid and Zantac), Vicks Inhaler

Sample Dialogue: Drug Testing Protocol

TASKS 7.1 (INTRODUCING DRUG TESTING) AND 7.2 (GUIDELINES FOR COLLECTING URINE SPECIMENS)

Use *Caregiver Handout for Conducting Drug Screens* (Handout 7.1).

Therapist: Okay, today we are going to go over how to collect urine drug screens and alcohol breath scans and some of the rules for doing these.

Caregiver: So, how often do we have to get these?

Therapist: Well, it depends on what drugs we need to test for. Since Tony mostly uses marijuana, then we will probably be able to get by with testing once a week.

Caregiver: So you will get the screen every week, when we come to your office?

Therapist: I will start by doing the screens with you here in my office. I will show you how one is done today. Once you are understand how it works, I will give you supplies, and you will be able to do these at home.

Tony: What? You gotta be kidding me.

Therapist: No, I'm serious.

Tony: How's she gonna do that?

Therapist: Good question—let's go over these handouts that I have here, as they explain everything pretty well. [Gives each participant a copy of the *Caregiver Handout for Conducting Drug Screens* (Handout 7.1).]

Caregiver: I see a lot of information here about drug screens. What about alcohol? Is that something you can detect with urine?

Therapist: That's a good question. The easiest way to test for alcohol is to use some disposable breath scans that we have available here at the office. I will show you how to use those too.

Caregiver: Okay, so let's see those drug cups.

Therapist: Here is a cup. Now, let's read over this handout (7.1) together carefully as it tells us exactly what we need to do. [Reads over Handout 7.1 with Tony and his mother while showing them the drug screen cups they will use.]

Tony: I hope you don't expect me to give you a sample today.

Caregiver: Why not?

Tony: You know it's going to be dirty. We already talked about me smoking with John last weekend, when we did stuff with triggers and planning a few minutes ago.

Therapist: That's okay. We still need to do one today so that your mom can practice. Also starting today the reward menu we made last week will go into effect.

Tony: So now I have to start earning everything?

Caregiver: Yep, no more free lunch.

Tony: Well, I don't have to go right now.

Therapist: How about if you go grab a drink? I'll buy you a soda, because I really appreciate how hard you have been trying and how cooperative you have been with all of this. Here is some change. The machine is down the hall.

Tony: So you are bribing me?

Therapist: No, I am rewarding you. The soda is to thank you for the hard work you have done so far. I know it is hard to sit here and tell us everything about your friends and drug use and I think you are doing a good job. Plus, I think it may help with your next task.

[Tony leaves the session temporarily.]

Therapist: Okay, Ms. Smith, while Tony is away, let's decide when you will collect the next screen.

Caregiver: So he's not supposed to know?

Therapist: Right. It's important that the screens be random and unexpected as that gives us the best chance of knowing if he has used or not. Usually we try to collect the screens within a day or so of a high-risk time.

Caregiver: Well, today is Monday. We know that weekends are the highest risk time for Tony. How about if I collect another screen next Sunday morning?

Therapist: That sounds like a good plan.

Caregiver: What if I have questions? This seems sort of complicated.

Therapist: Well, let me give you my work cell phone number. I'll be around Sunday morning. You can call me anytime between 10:00 A.M. and 9:00 P.M. if you have problems. Also, you will be in next Tuesday, so we can always test again Tuesday if we need to.

Caregiver: So am I supposed to clear out my bathroom at home, tape things up like it says on this handout?

Therapist: You have a choice. If you are comfortable watching Tony urinate into the cup, to make sure that he gives a clean sample, then you don't really need to take all of the steps on that sheet. If you feel more comfortable giving him some privacy, then following the steps on the handout is important as we need to make sure the sample is a good one.

Caregiver: Well, I can either follow the steps or get his stepfather to watch him. That would probably make the most sense.

Therapist: Yes, that sounds like a good plan.

[Tony returns to the session.]

Tony: Okay, I'm back.

Therapist: Are you ready to try?

Tony: I guess.

Therapist: Let's walk down the hall together. There is a bathroom here that is set up for this purpose. Tony, I need for you to take off your jacket and turn your pockets out for me.

Tony: Man, you don't trust me?

Therapist: Well, you are earning our trust with clean screens. My experience tells me that we need to do this, just to make sure. Drugs can have a weird effect on people. Drugs can make good people do bad things, like lie.

Tony: Not me.

Therapist: Glad to hear that. Now please turn your pants pockets out. [Goes through protocol with Tony while his mother observes the process. The urine screen results are positive for marijuana.]

Tony: Well, I told you it would be dirty.

Therapist: Yes, and we appreciate your honesty. In fact, in the future if you are dirty and tell us so, we may decide not to screen you. Instead, we can just mark you down for dirty in the checkbook.

Tony: Okay, that would make sense.

Caregiver: Is there any reason that I should screen him, even if he says he is dirty?

Therapist: Well, you might want to screen if you think he could be dirty for something else other than marijuana. As you have seen, the cups we have can screen for cocaine and amphetamines as well. We also have some cups here that screen for those three things plus methamphetamine, which is crystal meth, plus opiates like heroin and benzodiazepines like valium.

Caregiver: Well, I am more worried about alcohol.

Therapist: Okay. Why don't we agree that every once and awhile, just to be safe, one of us will give Tony the six-test drug cup just to be sure.

Tony: Man, you guys really don't trust me. I don't do that hard stuff.

Therapist: Well, Tony, using drugs can be dangerous. Sometimes people put things in the drugs that the user is not aware of. They may lace the blunt with cocaine or other things.

Tony: Not my sources. I have good contacts.

Therapist: Well, that may be true. But as I said earlier, drug use sometimes leads even good people to make bad decisions and to do mean things they wouldn't ordinarily do.

Tony: Man, you guys are paranoid.

Therapist: Well, I just see a lot of bad stuff in my line of work.

Caregiver: What about the test results? What do we do with that information?

Therapist: Well, what normally happens is that we go over the results with Tony, do an ABC assessment with him to find out what his triggers were and what exactly happened, then we help him modify his self-management plan and decide how he can avoid drug use next time.

Tony: We already did that earlier today, before we did all the urine screen stuff.

Therapist: Right. So we sort of did things backward today. Before we forget, let's both write down the results of this test (dirty) in your checkbook. I'll keep mine in my chart and you can take yours home.

Caregiver: Okay. Now that we have done that, I can see that we are almost out of time. Can you tell me about the breath scans?

Therapist: Good point. Let's do that now.

TASK 7.3: GUIDELINES FOR COLLECTING ALCOHOL BREATH SPECIMENS (AS NEEDED)

Use *Caregiver Handout for Collecting Alcohol Breath Specimens* (Handout 7.3)]

Therapist: Here is a breath scan tube. [Hands a tube to caregiver and one to Tony.] Let's look at the handout (7.3) and read about what to do.

Tony: Do I have to do one of these today? I almost never drink. This is stupid.

Caregiver: I think sometimes you drink when you have been smoking. Plus, I know when I was younger alcohol was a big deal.

Therapist: Tony, I know you have not been drinking today and I appreciate your patience with all of this testing. I can do the breath test on myself today to show your mom how it works.

Tony: Sounds good.

[Therapist goes through the protocol while his mother and Tony observe the process.]

Caregiver: Okay, so when do I do this?

Therapist: Well, you have to gather a breath scan while the person still has significant levels of alcohol in his or her body. The amount of time for detection varies from person to person depending on a lot of things, including how much the person had to drink and how fast his or her body metabolizes alcohol.

Caregiver: So I need to get it when Tony comes home from a place where he may have used?

Therapist: Correct. For example, once Tony has earned the ability to drive the car as his MVP, you will want to get a breath scan from him when he gets home that night.

Caregiver: What if it shows alcohol?

Therapist: Then we treat it just like a dirty urine screen. Tony would lose his MVP and not get points that week.

Caregiver: That would make sense. So, for instance, I might get a breath scan on Saturday night when he gets in from using the car. If that is clean, what about the urine drug screen?

Therapist: Many people like to get the drug screen at the same time. This way, you know if Tony has earned his MVP for the week and if you should give him points.

Caregiver: That makes sense. So I test him all at once and if the screens are clean for everything, he gets his MVP and points?

Therapist: Right.

Caregiver: What if he tests clean on Saturday, but I think he may be high on Monday?

Therapist: Good question. You would test him again on Monday, and if the result is dirty, you would take away the MVP.

Tony: What about the points?

Therapist: Well, your mom would probably want to call me if that happened. We may need to subtract some points for the dirty screen. What we usually do is decide how many screens we plan to give at the start of the week, then divide the number of points (12 in Level 1) by the number of screens.

Caregiver: So, if I plan to test Tony twice a week, while he is in Level 1, I will give him 12 divided by 2, or 6, points for each clean screen that week.

Therapist: Correct, and he can have his MVP if his last screen was clean. So, since Tony's MVP is using the car, he can only use the car when his last screen is clean.

Caregiver: Got it.

Tony: Can we go?

Therapist: Well, I think we have accomplished a lot with this session. Tony, thanks for being so cooperative. I believe you are going to do a good job following your plans this week. Remember the self-management plans we talked about at the first of the session?

Tony: Yes, I got it.

Therapist: Good, Ms. Smith, please feel free to call me if you have any questions this week. Tony, you can call too.

Caregiver: See you next Tuesday.

Therapist: Don't forget these cups and breath scans. I look forward to meeting with you both next week to see what progress you have made.

CHAPTER 8

Synthesizing the Components of Contingency Management

THERAPIST GOALS

1. **Conduct comprehensive sessions with the youth and family that combine all components of CM.**
2. **As CM therapy draws to a close, help the family develop a plan to continue assessing for potential drug use and maintaining the incentive system after treatment ends.**

OVERVIEW OF A COMPREHENSIVE CM SESSION

After youth and caregivers have practiced the central components of CM, therapists begin to integrate them into each treatment session. This chapter provides a guide for combining the behavioral (drug screens, contract, and reward menu) and cognitive-behavioral (ABC assessment, self-management planning, and drug refusal skills) aspects of CM as treatment progresses. Also, several strategies are described to help youth and families sustain clinical gains after the conclusion of treatment.

The Structure of Treatment over Time

The CM intervention protocol is generally applied in a straightforward manner that follows the sequence of chapters, but the timing and duration of treatment and the frequency of sessions can be adapted to youth and family needs. Optimally, after families have practiced each component of CM and the framework of a contract and reward menu is in place, subsequent sessions entail an integrated approach in which the CM components are reviewed and modified as needed. These sessions are usually used to monitor and adjust ongoing behavioral (e.g., reward menu) or cognitive-behavioral (e.g., self-management plans) aspects of treatment based on outcomes (e.g., dirty screen, difficulty implementing drug refusal skills). The end phase of treatment is typically signaled when the youth has remained abstinent from substance use for 8 consecutive weeks. At this point, the youth will be in Level II of the point-and-level reward system and ready to enter the maintenance phase (Level III) after 2 more sequential weeks of clean screens. Hence, the focus of these latter sessions shifts to the development of plans to maintain positive gains through continued monitoring of possible drug use and providing rewards for abstinence after treatment ends.

A Typical CM Session—after All Components of CM Have Been Introduced

Several benchmarks in treatment denote that a family has been oriented to CM well enough to move into sessions that combine all aspects of CM. These include the presence of:

1. A signed contract.
2. A reward menu.
3. Completed ABC assessments.
4. Completed self-management plans.
5. Recent drug testing and alcohol breath scan results.

When these aspects of treatment are in place, a typical session will encompass each component as outlined next.

Monitoring Drug Use

The therapist often starts the session by ensuring that a recent drug test has been appropriately collected. If a screen has not been provided in an appropriate time window, the therapist and caregiver obtain a test during the session. This procedure presents the therapist with an opportunity to address any difficulties the family might have encountered regarding drug screen collection, interpretation, or youth behavior related to the process. Monitoring substance use is a critical component of CM and serves as the foundation for the rest of the session. Note that because alcohol breath scans must be collected very close in time to alcohol use, breath scans obtained in a therapist's office will likely be negative (clean) regardless of use. Hence, if alcohol is a substance of abuse by the youth, missed breath scans should be counted as dirty, and the therapist should problem solve with caregivers to ensure the collection of valid screens during the forthcoming week.

Point-and-Level Reward System with Checkbook

Next, the therapist and family make an entry into the youth's checkbook based on the results of the drug and alcohol tests. The therapist takes this time to ensure that the behavioral plan outlined in the *Reward Menu* (Form 6.3) is being closely followed and helps the family adjust the plan if indicated. Care is taken to encourage families to remain hopeful and to view dirty screens as learning opportunities.

The ABC Assessment

After the behavioral aspects of CM have been addressed (i.e., test results, reward plan), the therapist asks the youth and caregiver to help determine the circumstances associated with the drug screen results. Working from the client's existing *ABC Assessment* (Form 4.2) and *Discovering Triggers of Your Substance Use* (Form 4.1) worksheets, the therapist helps the family complete a new *ABC Assessment* (Form 4.2) worksheet based on the youth's recent incident of substance use or, if the youth was clean, nonuse. The goal is to gain an understanding of what went wrong as well as what went right during the prior week regarding drug use triggers and the ways they were managed by the youth and family.

Developing Skills

Finally, the therapist, youth, and family work to modify the existing self-management plan, taking the new information into account. The therapist collaborates with the youth to write up a new *Self-Management Planning* (Form 5.1) worksheet that has been modified to address new triggers or difficulties that were identified. Even if the youth has been successful in maintaining abstinence the prior week, the family often needs to adjust the existing self-management plans for new triggers or situations that might cause difficulties. The therapist, youth, and caregiver use time during the session to role-play the self-management strategies and practice drug refusal skills if indicated.

OVERVIEW OF A CM SESSION NEAR THE END OF TREATMENT

The length of CM treatment will vary from youth to youth depending on factors such as therapist experience with CM, knowledge and capacity to engage key participants, the frequency and quality of sessions, whether sessions are provided in the home or office, caregiver ability to attend and participate in sessions, family capacity to impact peer and school drivers of substance abuse, and the youth's engagement in treatment. Our clinical experience indicates that there is no one typical trajectory or path that most youth follow to success. Rather, some teens respond almost immediately while others have frequent setbacks and take longer to get clean. As a result, CM is structured around meeting specific goals rather than completing therapy on a fixed timeline. These goals center on achieving drug abstinence as evidenced by results from substance use testing. In general, therapists have found that once a youth has managed to be free from drugs and alcohol for 8 weeks in a row (mid-Level II of the point-and-level reward system), he or she will soon be ready to enter the maintenance phase of the reward system (Level III; see *Point-and-Level System at a Glance* [Handout 6.1]), and planning should begin for sustaining abstinence after the end of treatment.

A Typical CM Session—Near the End of Treatment

The primary benchmark for determining that a youth and family are nearing the end of CM treatment is when the youth has obtained 8 straight weeks of clean drug screens and breath scans. At this point, the therapist modifies his or her clinical approach to anticipate entry into the maintenance phase, or Level III of the reward system (see *Point-and-Level System at a Glance* [Handout 6.1]). A typical session at this latter stage of treatment *still encompasses all the usual aspects of CM* as described previously, yet will also contain some new elements as outlined next.

The ABC Assessment

The therapist uses the ABC assessment component of CM as the vehicle for reviewing the triggers of drug use and abstinence and discussing key factors within the youth's social network (e.g., new prosocial friends, better parental monitoring, constructive goals) that are helping to sustain sobriety.

Developing Skills

While going over the youth's self-management plans and drug refusal skills, the therapist focuses on the broader picture and asks the family what types of skills will be needed in the future to sustain sobriety. Hence, the therapist helps the caregivers and youth to start anticipating the end of CM treatment and planning for how they will manage situations that will arise and place the youth at risk for relapse after treatment is concluded.

Monitoring Drug Use

As families begin to think about how they will help their youth stay clean from drugs after treatment ends, the therapist tries to persuade caregivers to continue monitoring the youth for substance use, albeit less frequently than during treatment. Hence, therapists help caregivers plan the specifics of when to screen their youth (e.g., Friday nights, intoxicated behavior) and what methods to use (e.g., test from drug store, smell of alcohol on breath). This is a good point in treatment to help the caregivers identify and obtain their own supply of urine drug cups and breath scans if they have not already done so. Therapists often help families find cups at local drug stores or use the *Drug and Alcohol*

Testing Resource List (Handout 7.2) to link them with Internet resources. Caregivers should have their own supply of drug testing materials and be familiar with their use before treatment ends.

Point-and-Level Reward System with Checkbook

Finally, the therapist works with family members to create a reward system to use after the youth has achieved 10 straight weeks of clean screens and, hence, completes Level II of the point-and-level reward system (see *Point-and-Level System at a Glance* [Handout 6.1]). The goal is to have a plan in place by the time the youth completes Level II. In general, therapists help families create a simpler version of the reward menu that relies solely on family resources and privileges for use in Level III as treatment ends. For instance, most families find it very helpful to continue to tie an MVP to the youth's sobriety. Hence, families need to make clear to the youth that substance use testing and associated consequences will continue after formal treatment with the therapist ends.

The End of Treatment

In general, CM treatment is complete after the youth has entered Level III of the point-and-level reward system and the family has a clear plan to continue to monitor the youth for drug use, reward abstinence, and address substance use. Ideally, caregivers will be able to generalize the ABC assessment and self-management planning skills taught by the therapist as well. Therapists often keep families in treatment a few weeks after they enter Level III to help problem solve any difficulties that might arise as the family shifts to more independent work. Some therapists like to maintain phone contact for a few more weeks to help ensure a successful transition.

Aims and Time Frame of the Following Tasks

The primary goal of the first task outlined in this chapter is for therapists to conduct treatment sessions that integrate all the CM components. This task is the goal of all sessions that occur after the components of CM have been introduced. The second task is for therapists to help families plan for the end of treatment by developing maintenance strategies that can be used by families to sustain treatment gains. Therapists usually complete sessions during these phases of treatment in an hour.

THERAPIST TASK 8.1: CONDUCTING AN INTEGRATED CM SESSION

Objective

1. Conduct a comprehensive session with the youth and family that combines all components of CM.

Materials

- *Therapist Checklist 8.1: Conducting an Integrated CM Session*
- Youth's *Reward Menu* (Form 6.3)
- Youth's *Checkbook* (Form 6.4)
- Youth's *ABC Assessment* (Form 4.2)
- Youth's *Self-Management Planning* (Form 5.1)

Accomplishing the Objective

The goal of the session is for each of the components of CM to be addressed in an integrated manner.

Monitoring Drug Use

The therapist frequently starts the session by determining the results of the last urine drug screen and alcohol breath scan obtained from the youth. If a recent test is not available, or if family members experienced difficulty or uncertainty about test results, the therapist and caregiver collect another test.

Point-and-Level Reward System with Checkbook

Following the steps outlined in *Therapist Checklist 8.1: Conducting an Integrated CM Session*, the therapist works with the youth and caregiver to make appropriate entries into the youth's *Checkbook* (Form 6.4) and to ensure that the behavioral plan outlined in the *Reward Menu* (Form 6.3) is being closely followed. Any adjustments that are needed to make the rewards more salient or to problem solve difficulties are done at this time. Behavioral plans are often a work in progress and normally require some modification.

ABC Assessment

After the more behavioral aspects of CM (drug testing, reward menu) have been addressed, the therapist examines the reasons for the youth's success or lack of success in gaining or sustaining abstinence. Using the youth's completed *ABC Assessment* (Form 4.2) worksheets, the therapist reviews what might be different since the last session and helps the family complete a new *ABC Assessment* (Form 4.2) based on this new information. If the youth's screen was dirty, the focus is on the ABCs of the drug use. If the screen was clean, the therapist helps the youth recall a situation during the prior week in which he or she was presented with the opportunity to use substances and did not. Then, an ABC assessment is completed with nonuse as the focal point rather than substance use. That is, the youth delineates the antecedents, behaviors, and consequences that accompanied his or her decision to not use drugs.

Developing Skills

Next, the therapist works with the family to review the previously completed *Self-Management Planning* (Form 5.1) worksheet and to create new plans based on the relevant information obtained during the current session. The therapist then role-plays the plans with the youth and caregiver and helps the youth practice drug refusal skills.

Assigning Homework

As a last step, the therapist assigns appropriate homework. Homework assignments will vary from client to client, but often include having the caregiver collect a urine drug screen or breath scan at home and getting family members to help the youth practice or carry out self-management strategies. Having families work together on aspects of CM treatment outside of treatment sessions plays an integral role in accelerating and maintaining treatment gains.

THERAPIST TASK 8.2: CONDUCTING AN INTEGRATED CM SESSION NEAR THE END OF TREATMENT

Objective

1. Conduct sessions near the end of treatment that will help the family develop a plan to continue to assess for potential drug use and maintain the incentive system after treatment ends.

Materials

- *Therapist Checklist 8.2: Conducting an Integrated CM Session near the End of Treatment*
- Youth's *Reward Menu* (Form 6.3)
- Youth's *Checkbook* (Form 6.4)
- Youth's *ABC Assessment* (Form 4.2)
- Youth's *Self-Management Planning* (Form 5.1)

Accomplishing the Objective

The broad goal is to prepare the youth and caregivers to sustain treatment gains after therapy ends. Thus, after youth have been abstinent for approximately 8 weeks in a row, therapists modify their treatment sessions to help families prepare for the completion of treatment. First, therapists can plan to have the family ready to implement a new family-based *Reward Menu* (Form 6.3) by the time the youth enters Level III of the point-and-level reward system (see *Point-and-Level System at a Glance* [Handout 6.1]), which occurs when he or she has been clean for 10 weeks in a row. Second, therapists can have the family practice implementing all aspects of treatment (i.e., new reward menu, family-based drug testing) with increasing independence such that they are ready to complete formal CM treatment within several weeks of entering Level III. A typical session at this stage *still encompasses all the usual aspects of CM* as described in Task 8.1, but also addresses the following elements over the next several sessions.

Review Success.

Following *Therapist Checklist 8.2: Conducting an Integrated CM Session near the End of Treatment,* the therapist reviews the success the youth is having in treatment and helps the family identify the key youth, family, peer, school, and community factors that contributed to this success. Often the therapist will use information from prior ABC assessments of failures and successes to help understand which factors put the youth at risk and which supported abstinence.

Predict the Youth and Family's Ability to Sustain Gains.

The therapist engenders hope in families while also noting the potential for relapse. Caregivers are reminded that both adults and adolescents who are trying to quit drugs, alcohol, or nicotine frequently have relapses. The next phase of treatment, therefore, aims to help family members plan their response if drug use should recur. A focus on the gains the youth has made and the family's role in these gains is central to this objective.

Put Plans into Place for Sustaining Abstinence and Dealing with Relapse.

Building on the work the youth and family accomplished previously with existing self-management plans and drug refusal skill sets, the therapist and family identify what skills will be needed to help the youth sustain abstinence after therapy has ended. To the extent that these skills require further development, the therapist pursues this course. Over the next several sessions, families create concrete plans that are detailed on new *Self-Management Planning* (Form 5.1) worksheets. These plans are implemented and modified during the final weeks of treatment such that families have a practiced version they can follow when treatment ends.

Update the Reward Menu.

Form 6.3 is revised as the youth moves into Level III of the point-and-level system and the final phase of treatment. Using the most current version of the youth's *Reward Menu* (Form 6.3), the family is encouraged to either eliminate or modify rewards that have not been helpful. In turn, if the therapist has been providing rewards as incentives, the family should look for alternative reinforcers in the natural ecology that can substitute for these. In particular, the MVP should be examined closely to ensure its continued relevance to the youth and family. For example, if a youth has been rewarded for clean drug screens with cell phone access, the therapist should confirm that caregivers plan to continue to link cell phone usage with abstinence after treatment ends.

Develop a Plan for Continued Substance Testing.

Because families are urged to continue to monitor their youth's drug use, albeit at a potentially reduced rate, they require a method for obtaining drug tests and alcohol breath scans. The therapist helps families access their own supply of drug testing materials either through a local drug store or with telephone or web-based orders (*Drug and Alcohol Testing Resource List* [Handout 7.2]). Because caregivers must be capable of administering these tests on their own, testing materials should be obtained well before treatment ends to allow the therapist time to resolve problems that might develop. After the family has a method for testing, they will also need a plan for when to test. One rule of thumb is to continue to test youth at times of high risk for 6 to 12 months after treatment ends. This guideline is broad, and some youth might need more or less frequent testing depending on their histories of use, triggers, and the risk and protective factors inherent in their environments.

Create Criteria for Calling the Therapist or Returning to Therapy.

Finally, families should be provided with guidelines about what sorts of signs (e.g., multiple positive urine drug screens in spite of implementation of maintenance plan) and symptoms warrant calling the therapist or returning for treatment in the future. The therapist may want to schedule telephone follow-up calls during the first few weeks after treatment to check in with families and provide additional support or guidance if indicated.

THERAPIST CHECKLISTS FOR CHAPTER 8: SYNTHESIZING THE COMPONENTS OF CONTINGENCY MANAGEMENT

THERAPIST CHECKLIST 8.1

Conducting an Integrated CM Session

Case number: ______________ **Session date:** ______________

I have explained that (check each item covered in session):

___ Now that you have learned about the individual parts of CM, such as the ABC assessments, self-management plans, drug screens, and rewards, it is time to start putting all of these parts together each session.

___ For example, we will start sessions by looking at the results of the last drug screen/breath scan collected on (*youth's name*). If (*youth's name*) has not given a screen recently, we will collect one.

___ Then, based on the results of this screen, we will look at (*youth's name's*) checkbook and add points if they have been earned with a clean screen. We will confirm the loss of the MVP if the screen was dirty.

___ At this point in the session we will discuss the reward system. I will be checking to make sure that the system is working appropriately and answer any questions you may have.

___ If (*youth's name's*) most recent screen was clean, this may be a good time for him/her to buy items or privileges using the checkbook. I will also look over the checkbook, so please bring it with you each visit.

___ Then, based on the results of the most recent drug screen, we will complete a new *ABC Assessment* (Form 4.2) to help us understand the antecedents, behaviors, and consequences of either the most recent incident of drug use or a recent time that (*youth's name*) was able to avoid drug use.

___ Next, we will review (*youth's name's*) most recent self-management plans and adjust the *Self-Management Planning* worksheet (Form 5.1) to take the new information we have learned into account.

___ In other words, each week, (*youth's name*) will have a new set of plans for dealing with triggers that might occur. These plans will build on the plans from prior weeks based on whether they succeeded or failed.

___ Finally, I will give your family homework each week. Assignments will include, for example, collecting drug tests, practicing self-management plans and drug refusal skills, and thinking about the ABCs of drug use or nonuse that occur between sessions.

THERAPIST CHECKLIST 8.2

Conducting an Integrated CM Session near the End of Treatment

Case number: ______________ **Session date:** ______________

I have explained that (check each item covered in session):

___ Now that (*youth's name*) has been able to demonstrate tremendous success by being clean for 8 weeks in a row, it's time for us to start thinking about the next phase of treatment.

___ As you may remember (see *Point-and-Level System at a Glance* [Handout 6.1]), our current reward plan is scheduled to last until (*youth's name*) has been clean for 10 weeks in a row. At that point in time (*youth's name*) will enter into Level III of the reward system. This is a big accomplishment, and we will plan to have a celebration when (*youth's name*) has been clean for 10 weeks straight.

___ In the meantime, we need to think about how your family is going to help (*youth's name*) sustain his/her gains as we enter this final phase of treatment.

___ Let's start by trying to understand the successes so far. I'd like for you to give me some ideas about why you think (*youth's name*) has been able to stay clean. As we do this exercise, I'm going to look at the ABC assessments and self-management plans we have created together thus far. I want to make sure we take all of these into account.

[The therapist and family spend time developing consensus on the drivers to the youth's success.]

___ Now that we have a better understanding of why (*youth's name*) has been able to stay clean this long, it's time to talk about ways your family can work together to help (*youth's name*) continue to stay drug free.

___ It often helps if we spend some time creating some new *Self-Management Planning* worksheets (Form 5.1) for you to document how you plan to contribute to (*youth's name's*) continued efforts to stay clean during this last phase of treatment and after treatment ends.

[The therapist and family create and document new self-management strategies to help sustain gains.]

___ Good work. Our next task is to talk about ways your family can continue to track (*youth's name's*) progress. As you know from our experience together, getting off drugs can be really hard to do. As a result, we strongly encourage families to have a system in place to periodically monitor for drug use, even after therapy ends.

___ Let's talk about how you might be able to monitor (*youth's name*) for drug/alcohol use after treatment is over. I'd like to help you set up a very clear plan about when you will check to see if (*youth's name*) might have relapsed and how you will go about assessing this.

(cont.)

___ [The therapist develops and documents clear rules with the family concerning the frequency, conditions, and process of future drug testing.]

___ Now that we have a plan for testing in the future, we also need to set up a plan for rewarding (*youth's name*) as he continues to be successful staying away from drugs and alcohol.

___ I have copies of your most recent *Reward Menu* (Form 6.3) [passes copies to participants], and I would like us to look at this to help us decide what types of rewards have been working or not working for you.

[The therapist reviews successes and difficulties with the current reward system.]

___ Now, I'd like for us to create a new *Reward Menu* (Form 6.3) [passes blank forms to participant]. This one will be much like the last one, with the main difference being that all of the rewards will need to be items, activities, and privileges your family can provide.

___ Let's start with the MVP. This is often the most powerful part of the reward plan. We should look at the MVP you are providing now and decide if it makes sense to keep that one, change it, or totally replace it as we move into the last stage of treatment.

[The therapist and family decide on future MVP.]

___ Okay. The final stage of preparation involves deciding what other types of rewards you would like to tie to abstinence in the future. Now that you have an MVP in place and plan to always tie that to abstinence, are there other rewards you would like to put on this sheet to help show (*youth's name*) how much you appreciate his or her continued hard work in staying clean?

___ Some families like to continue to have a reward menu that is very much like the one we have been working from in which the youth earns weekly points and continues to buy rewards. This method requires continued weekly screens and is a safe way to help ensure the youth is closely monitored and well compensated.

___ Other families choose to develop a menu that is somewhat simpler than the current one. This menu continues to feature an MVP, yet the other items the youth earns can be given at various time intervals if he/she continues to stay clean. For instance, caregivers may decide that at the end of each week in which the youth has not demonstrated any symptoms of drug use, he/she may have one additional item or privilege from a list the family creates. Some families also like to tie bigger prizes to longer stretches of sobriety. For example, the youth may earn a larger prize after staying clean for another 2 months.

___ Note that regardless of the type of reward plan we create, you should continue to closely watch (*youth's name*) for signs and symptoms of substance use and follow the drug/alcohol testing schedule we created.

[The therapist and family develop a reward menu that meets the needs of the youth and is manageable for the family after the end of treatment.]

___ Congratulations! You now have a plan in place to help (*youth's name*) stay clean. Your family has done a good job putting this together, and I bet that you will continue to be successful.

(cont.)

___ For homework, I'd like for you all to read over the plans we just created and see if there is anything else we should add or change. Also, you will need to continue with your normal weekly work of gathering a random urine/alcohol screen and implementing the self-management plans.

___ In the next session we will review the plans we created today so that we can be ready to implement them as soon as (*youth's name*) reaches Level III of treatment.

___ As soon as (*youth's name*) reaches Level III of treatment, we will start to implement the new drug testing protocol, reward menu, and self-management plans. After you have had a chance to work out any concerns with those plans, we can set a date for treatment termination.

___ Your family is doing a fantastic job. I congratulate your hard work and predict that you will continue to do well.

Sample Dialogue: Synthesizing the Components of Contingency Management

TASK 8.1: CONDUCTING AN INTEGRATED CM SESSION

Therapist: Welcome, Tony, Ms. Smith, and Mr. Smith. It's nice to see you.

Stepfather: Remember, you can call me Al. I don't really like being so formal.

Therapist: Sure. That will make things easier. How is your family doing this week?

Caregiver: Well, it sort of hinges on Tony's drug screen results. One of the reasons Al came with me is that we can't agree on how to read the screens.

Tony: Yeah, Al just can't believe I might be clean.

Stepfather: I'll believe it when I see it.

Therapist: Tell me your concerns.

Stepfather: Well, we gave Tony a urine screen on Saturday after he came in from being out with his friends, just like you suggested.

Tony: I can't believe you guys thought I would drink or use drugs over at Shanda's house. I keep telling you she's straight.

Caregiver: We were just following the protocols, Tony, like we agreed in therapy.

Therapist: Good. So where did you run into problems?

Caregiver: Reading the test results. We're hoping you can help us understand how to read the results we got.

Tony: I keep telling you guys the test was clean, there was a line.

Stepfather: Yeah, but you could hardly see it. The tests on that cup for amphetamines and cocaine had two strong lines that were pretty dark, but the test for marijuana had a fainter line. So I was telling my wife that we should count the screen dirty.

Therapist: Well, I have to say that this is a very common question that a number of families have had. I apologize for not warning you that this may happen. Since this has come up before, I contacted the company to find out more about how to handle this. The appropriate response for a faint line is to count it as clean.

Tony: See? Told you!

Stepfather: Well, it looked like it was starting to go away, like it was reacting to something, so it seemed to me it should be counted dirty.

Therapist: I understand, yet what the company said when I called them is that the tests they provide are qualitative, not quantitative. What that means is that they aren't capable of being partially negative or partially positive. They are either dirty or clean, and *any* line, no matter how faint, should be interpreted as a clean screen.

Stepfather: Hmmm, still makes me suspicious.

Therapist: I understand that teens often lie to their parents when they are using drugs, and it's pretty common for parents to take some time before they start trusting their child again.

Caregiver: I think Tony really had a clean screen.

Therapist: You do?

Caregiver: Yes, the reason I think so is because I know he was trying to work the plan. He really wants to get the car this coming weekend, because of a school dance. He has been trying the self-management things we worked on, and I think he has managed to avoid John the last couple of weeks.

Stepfather: Well, maybe. I think the new girl he's interested in doesn't use.

Tony: How about if I take the test again?

Therapist: We can do that if you like. Yet we need to agree now that a faint line will be interpreted as clean.

Stepfather: No, I'm okay going with clean this time.

Therapist: Okay. It may also help if you guys are careful to follow the handout I gave you. Make sure the test is either random or after a time that you're most worried Tony may have used. Another thing parents sometimes do if they are concerned is to get the screen first thing in the morning. Drugs tend to be concentrated in the urine then.

Caregiver: So now what do we do?

Therapist: Well, I want to congratulate Tony for having a clean screen.

Tony: Doesn't feel like congratulations. You guys don't trust me.

Therapist: It takes time to earn back trust. You made a great start this week with a clean screen.

Tony: [Appears dissatisfied.] I dunno.

Therapist: This is a good time to give you the points you earned. Did you bring your checkbook?

Caregiver: Oh, we forgot.

Therapist: That's okay. I have a copy of his checkbook here. I'm going to step out for a minute and make you a copy. [Returns and hands checkbook account sheet to Ms. Smith.] I also copied Tony's most recent reward menu, ABC assessments, and self-management plans. We'll be looking these over in a few minutes.

Caregiver: What next?

Therapist: Well, now is a good time for you to give Tony his points. Why don't you add them to the balance in his checkbook?

Caregiver: What do I write?

Therapist: Well, you may want to put the date and "clean screen," then add the 12 points.

Caregiver: So that brings him to 37 points because this is his first clean screen.

Tony: How about my MVP? I would like the car keys, please.

Stepfather: Wait a minute, not so fast.

Caregiver: We agreed that you can have the car this Saturday until 9 P.M. for an approved activity with approved people.

Tony: Sounds good.

Stepfather: How do we know he won't go out and use?

Tony: You can test me when I come home.

Caregiver: That is correct. I plan to do a breath scan and a drug screen on Tony when he brings the car back Saturday night, like I tested him last weekend.

Stepfather: Just plan to use your mother's car.

Therapist: You all are doing a nice job. It's important that Tony gets the reward you promised because a well-chosen MVP can be very motivating.

Caregiver: As you can see, Tony is motivated to drive.

Therapist: What about points? I was wondering if Tony might be interested in spending some points. He can spend some, or even all, of his points now since his last screen was clean.

Tony: I'm saving up for the iPod.

Therapist: Looking at your reward menu, I see that the iPod will cost 50 points. It looks like you are halfway there.

Stepfather: That sounds expensive.

Caregiver: This is a Shuffle; it's less expensive than most, and I promised Tony he could have one if he earned it.

Therapist: I wonder if we might need to go over the list with you more in-depth, Al, to make sure we are all on the same page?

Stepfather: No, my wife went over it with me. I'm okay with everything on here.

Caregiver: I had to make Tony do his laundry last week.

Therapist: I was going to ask about that. Sounds like Tony must have failed to attend school all 5 days.

Caregiver: He went 4 days, but insisted he was sick Thursday, and I know he was well enough to go.

Therapist: So you withheld doing the laundry?

Tony: I had to do it myself, Sunday.

Stepfather: He turned his socks pink by washing them with his red basketball jersey. It was pretty funny.

Tony: Want me to do your laundry?

Therapist: All right, so I'm going to check off that you guys are doing a good job with both the drug testing and the reward menu part of therapy. Now I'd like for us to look at Tony's last clean drug screen and do an ABC assessment of nonuse.

Caregiver: We usually do this on drug use, not nonuse.

Therapist: Right. We'll apply the same principles, only focus on Tony not using. [Passes out Tony's latest ABC assessment and a blank form.] Okay, Tony, can you think of a specific time last week when you almost used drugs or were really tempted to use?

Tony: Okay, well, hmmm, last week, I was standing outside the gym after practice, waiting for my mom to pick me up. It was getting dark, and I saw John's friend Derrick over in the smoking area. He motioned to me and I was about to walk over to talk to him, which would have made it likely that I might use or at least be tempted to buy some pot. Then one of the other guys on the team, Leon, came over. I decided to talk to him for a few minutes instead. As we were talking, my mom drove up. So I guess hanging with Leon, then my mom arriving on time, helped me not to use.

Therapist: All right, so let's think of some of the antecedents, or triggers, of nondrug use.

Tony: Well, one trigger was basketball. I always feel good about myself and healthy after I play ball. So, when I saw Derrick, I thought "Oh no, I hope he doesn't ask me to use" instead of thinking "Oh boy, I hope he has some."

Therapist: Okay, what else?

Tony: Well, Leon being there probably helped. He's straight and wouldn't approve of me smoking weed. Oh, and my mom being on time, that helped.

Therapist: Good. I am writing those triggers or antecedents down. Now, what behaviors did you exhibit to keep from using?

Tony: Well, I stayed put. I didn't walk over to meet Derrick. I also sort of didn't look at him much, I kind of ignored him. Also, I made a point of talking to Leon, trying to keep him there to talk to me until my mom came.

Therapist: Great. Now, what sort of consequences did this incident of nonuse have?

Tony: I get the car this weekend, and I have some points.

Caregiver: And I am proud of you. Al and I are both proud.

Therapist: Good job. Now we need to look at Tony's self-management plan and decide if there are things about the plan that need to be tweaked or changed to take advantage of this new information we've collected.

Stepfather: Seems like Tony should stay away from the smoking area.

Tony: Yeah, I think next time I'll wait in the gym. That way I won't see my friends in the smoking pit.

Therapist: What else?

Tony: Well, I can hang with Leon and some guys on the team more. They're busy practicing so they don't smoke as much as my friends.

Caregiver: That sounds like a good idea. I was also thinking, you have a cell phone now, you could call me and talk to me if you need. That would make you look busy and maybe you could avoid talking to the smokers that way.

Therapist: Okay. I am adding these tactics to your set of self-management strategies. Let's keep brainstorming for a few minutes, then we'll grade these and decide which ones Tony might plan to use. [Works with the family to get modified plans in place.]

Stepfather: Well, we have to run. I need to head into work tonight.

Therapist: Yes, time is up.

Caregiver: Do we do the usual homework?

Therapist: Yes, I almost forgot. I believe the plan is for you both to allow Tony to use the car this Saturday. Then, when he comes home, you will give him a breath scan and drug screen. You will record the results in the checkbook and bring the checkbook to your session next week.

Stepfather: What about the plans?

Therapist: You're ahead of me and you are correct. The other homework is for Tony and your family to implement the self-management plans. As you can see from this week's example, you, as parents, are an important part of Tony's plans. Notice that Ms. Smith arriving at the gym on time to pick up Tony had a big impact on his ability to remain drug free this week. I'll see you guys next week.

TASKS 8.2: CONDUCTING AN INTEGRATED CM SESSION NEAR THE END OF TREATMENT

Therapist: Welcome! I'm glad you both could make it today. Where's Al?

Caregiver: He couldn't make it today, too much work.

Tony: I tested clean again.

Therapist: Fantastic. Let's write that down. I've got my version of Tony's checkbook ledger. Do you have yours?

Tony: Yeah, I had to run back in the house and grab it.

Caregiver: It's already done. I added Tony's 25 points on Saturday night, when he tested clean. His breath scan was clean too.

Therapist: Let's count the number of weeks you've had a clean screen and scan.

Tony: I know it off the top of my head: It's 8. I've been clean for 8 weeks in a row.

Therapist: Wow, that's fantastic. Do you know what that means?

Tony: That I get to buy some more stuff?

Therapist: Well, yes, it means that, but it also signals to me that it is time for us to start planning for your transition to Level III, our highest and last level of treatment.

Tony: So am I getting close to being done?

Therapist: If you are able to stay clean for 2 more weeks, then you will move to Level III. We often work with families for another 2 to 4 weeks once they get to Level III, just to make sure they don't have any questions or problems. Then they graduate.

Tony: Hmm, I like the idea of having more free time, but does that mean I won't get stuff anymore?

Therapist: That is a good question, because it leads right into the topic of our session. The primary goal of our session this week, and probably next week as well, will be to help you and your family figure out how to help you maintain these great gains that you have all made.

Tony: I'm good as long as I keep getting the car.

Therapist: Great. I'll keep that in mind. First, before we talk about the car, I'd like to think back about your success with you and your mom. I'd like for both of you to identify the biggest drivers or causes for you being able to get clean and stay clean.

Caregiver: Well, Al and I have been watching Tony better. We don't give him as much freedom as we used to, and we try to know where he is and who he's with all the time.

Therapist: I cannot applaud you enough for that. Parental supervision and monitoring of their teens is the best way to help kids stay away from drugs. What else?

Tony: John, taking John out of the picture really helped.

Therapist: Right, you learned to avoid him and . . .

Caregiver: John went to a juvenile rehabilitation center upstate, and that really helped.

Therapist: Okay, good point. So we need to make sure your family has a plan to put into place when he returns.

Tony: Maybe, but I'm playing basketball now and my girlfriend hates drugs and most of the guys on the basketball team don't use, or don't use like my old friends did.

Therapist: You changed your friend group. That can be a very powerful way to avoid drugs. From what you've told me over the last few months, you've moved away from friends who use and started gaining friends who don't use. Bravo! That can be hard to do.

Caregiver: Yes, I'm starting to realize how important his friends can be.

Therapist: While you guys have mentioned some of the biggest drivers to success, I think there are probably some more. I'd like to look over the ABC assessments that we completed together concerning both use and nonuse. Let's see if there are other ways you've overcome your triggers. [With the family, spends time developing consensus on the drivers of the youth's success and identifying potential concerns for the future.] So, to summarize, you both feel that to help Tony be successful in the future, your family should continue to monitor him closely, meet his friends, support his participation in organized sports, enforce rules for school attendance and performance, and help him stay away from peers who use. You both felt that Tony would be most likely to have problems in the future when John returns from placement and when basketball is over. That sounds right on target.

Tony: Now what?

Therapist: Let's look at your most recent self-management plans and think about how you will work to sustain your current level of success. In particular, let's make sure we develop plans to deal with John coming back into town and the basketball season ending. [With family, creates and documents new self-management strategies targeting maintenance and the end of treatment.] Great work. It looks like you both have some good ideas for dealing with John when he shows back up, and I'm glad Tony will be able to start working at his uncle's trucking transport garage when basketball season is over. That should help Tony stay busy and avoid drugs.

Tony: And earn money. I really want to earn money.

Caregiver: Yes, you will earn money, but we're going to put most of it in the bank. Then you can have a real checking account instead of this fake one.

Therapist: Right, and we talked about monitoring Tony's money as that can often trigger drug use as well.

Caregiver: I feel like I have a grip on the triggers and self-management plans. What I'm wondering about is the drug testing. Do we still drug test Tony once we are in Level III?

Therapist: Yes, we do. There are two differences about testing in Level III. One is that we may not test as often. The three of us and your husband will need to think about how often Tony should be tested and under what conditions. It will be important to keep testing Tony from time to time as you are still going to want to link rewards and privileges to Tony's continued abstinence. The other difference is that we'll need to help you obtain your own testing cups. They have cups at the local drug store. Also I have a list of potential mail order resources I can share with you.

Caregiver: Are they expensive?

Therapist: I can help you find some that are less than $10 a cup.

Caregiver: That can still add up. How often do you think we'll have to test?

Therapist: There are lots of approaches to this, and it largely depends on how well Tony is doing. Many families start by testing every week, then move to testing less frequently, and finally just if the youth shows signs of drug use or has recently been in a high-risk situation.

Caregiver: Well, since Tony is probably going to continue to want to drive, I feel like we should test him once a week at first.

Tony: Ah, Mom, why don't you trust me?

Caregiver: I am starting to trust you again, Tony. I just think it may help if you know we're really going to keep watching you for awhile, even when treatment is over.

Therapist: I like your way of thinking. Why don't you go home and talk to Mr. Smith about the testing schedule this week. We'll try to finalize it next week. It would be good if your husband could come.

Caregiver: Yes, we'll want to get his opinion. He's going to be nervous about treatment ending.

Therapist: Great. Also, could you look in your local drug store and price the marijuana testing cups this week? I have a resource sheet as well that you might find helpful. [Gives caregiver a copy of *Drug and Alcohol Testing Resource List* (Handout 7.2).] It would help if you could look up a few of these sites or call the phone numbers and see what the prices of their cups are.

Caregiver: How long will we need to keep this up?

Therapist: Well, that can really vary. Most families try to keep testing their child periodically until they've been clean for at least 6 months. Some like to go longer, approaching a year. I think the key is to be watching for the signs that problems are reemerging and then test if those show up.

Therapist: This leads me to the final part of Tony's maintenance plan that we need to discuss today. We need to help create a new reward menu for Tony.

Tony: Why?

Therapist: Well, I have a couple of reasons. First, there may be things on your reward menu that no longer interest you. It is often helpful to redo these every few weeks to make sure you have rewards you really want to work toward. Second, pretty soon you will graduate from CM, so we need a reward menu that doesn't have rewards that come from the clinic or me on it anywhere.

Caregiver: Okay, I have Tony's current reward menu here in front of me. In what ways do we need to change it?

Therapist: Good question. Let's look it over and decide, starting with the MVP. [with the family, decides on an appropriate MVP, reviews the reward menu for success or problems, and generates a new reward menu.]

Tony: Are we done?

Therapist: Yes, that's enough for this week. I want to congratulate you both. Your family did a fantastic job.

Tony: Thanks. See you next week.

Therapist: Just one more minute. Let's review the homework. [Reviews assignments with the family.]

Caregiver: I'll do my best to get Al to come. I think he needs to be here for this part.

Therapist: I agree. Please call me if we need to schedule at a different time so that Al can make the meeting.

Caregiver: I will.

Therapist: Have a good week.

CHAPTER 9

Conducting Contingency Management without Caregivers

THERAPIST GOALS

1. **Conduct productive CM sessions with the youth when caregivers have missed particular sessions.**
2. **Conduct CM treatment with the adolescent with minimal or no caregiver support.**

OVERVIEW OF IMPLEMENTING CM WITHOUT CAREGIVERS

Research data strongly support the implementation of CM techniques in the context of the parent–child relationship. As described previously, adolescent drug use is largely driven by contextual factors that caregivers are responsible for managing (deviant peer affiliation, family conflict, poor parental monitoring, school problems). Drug use interventions are most likely to be effective when they can impact these contextual drivers of youth drug use. The CM interventions described in this book rely on developing the caregiver's ability to modify the youth's environment such that abstinence is rewarded and drug use punished. Thus, attempting the intervention without caregiver involvement should be done only as a last resort, after all reasonable attempts have been made to engage caregivers and obtain other adult social support involvement.

Nevertheless, even when the therapist has gone to great lengths to cultivate engagement with a caregiver in CM treatment, it is possible that the caregiver will not be available for all treatment sessions or, in the worst case, that a caregiver might not participate in the treatment at all. The following suggestions are provided for managing the absence of the caregiver at particular points in the CM treatment process as well as for circumstances in which minimal caregiver support is forthcoming throughout treatment. Please note, however, if youth start treatment without a caregiver, the therapist should periodically attempt to bring the caregiver or other adult social support into the treatment to help attain and generalize therapeutic gains.

Determining the Need for Substance Use Treatment (Chapter 2)

If caregivers are absent from the initial assessment sessions, the following steps are recommended.

Explain to the Youth Why His or Her Drug Use Is a Problem.

Here the therapist should be prepared to give concrete examples of how drug use is contributing to problems identified by the referral source and youth. These examples should focus on things that have happened when the youth has used substances rather than on more abstract issues such as the youth's health or future well-being. The therapist might note, for example, that the youth gets in trouble for skipping school to smoke marijuana with his friends.

Determine Whether the Youth's Caregiver Knows or Suspects That the Youth Uses Drugs.

If the youth thinks the caregiver does not know or suspect his or her substance use, consider together how best to inform the caregiver. The therapist might have to be persistent and creative to cultivate the youth's willingness to inform the caregiver of the drug use. Federal regulations about the disclosure of client alcohol and drug use are extremely stringent. Therapists should follow agency policies regarding client confidentiality and the protections required by HIPAA. Because of federal regulations that protect clients specifically from unwanted disclosures of their alcohol or drug information, the therapist can share information about the youth's drug use with the caregiver only when the youth signs a consent form allowing such information sharing. If the youth is fearful of the caregiver's reaction, it might be helpful to role-play the session in which the adolescent tells the caregiver about his or her drug use. Alternatively, it might be preferable for the therapist to first meet alone with the caregiver (with the youth's consent) to help manage reactions such as alarm, anger, sadness, or feelings of betrayal.

Contact the Caregiver.

The caregiver can be contacted after the youth agrees to the plan. If the caregiver brings the youth to appointments, he or she can be asked to attend the youth's next appointment to discuss the next steps in the youth's treatment. If the youth's regular appointment time is not convenient for the caregiver, a more convenient time can be offered. If the caregiver does not bring the youth to treatment sessions, the therapist can make telephone contact with the caregiver to explain the reasons to meet together to discuss next steps in treatment.

ABC Assessment of Drug Use (Chapter 4)

For the following sections, recommendations are given for caregiver absences that are *temporary* (i.e., missing a limited number of sessions) or *permanent* (i.e., showing minimal presence or support of treatment).

Temporary Caregiver Absence

When a caregiver is absent from the initial session outlining the ABC assessment process, the therapist might be able to continue with the original goals of this session. Most of the steps required to implement the ABC assessment can be conducted in an individual format with the youth alone. The therapist can review and explain the content outlined in Chapter 4 and use the same session checklists and forms with the youth. However, the therapist conducting an individual session with the youth has several additional responsibilities. These include:

1. *Before* starting the individual session with the youth, the therapist emphasizes the important role of the youth's caregiver in the treatment process.

2. *During* the session, the therapist should refer to specific ways the caregiver will be involved in treatment. The therapist also asks the youth to give the caregiver blank copies of the *Discovering Triggers of Your Substance Use* (Form 4.1) and the *ABC Assessment* (Form 4.2) worksheets and to describe the use of these to the caregiver. The therapist might ask the youth to role-play the process of describing the forms to the caregiver.

3. *After* the session, the therapist should provide information to the caregiver about the ABC assessment process, ensure that the caregiver understands the process, and cultivate caregiver engagement. The therapist should schedule a call with the caregiver as quickly as possible to ensure that the caregiver understands and is willing to participate in the ABC assessment. Cultivating caregiver understanding is important for at least two reasons. First, the caregiver's support is needed to complete the homework assigned to the youth. Second, subsequent components of the CM protocol—self-management planning and the contingency management contract—build on the ABC assessment process. As noted previously, however, federal regulations about the disclosure of client alcohol and drug use are extremely stringent. Therapists should follow local, state, and federal policies regarding client confidentiality and the protections required by HIPAA.

When the caregiver attended the session that introduced the ABC assessment process, but was unable to attend subsequent sessions involving the ABC assessment, the therapist can call the caregiver before and after conducting an individual session with the youth. During the telephone conversation, the therapist should obtain the caregiver's perspective on the following issues.

1. *Youth's drug use.* The therapist asks the caregiver about whether and how often the youth has used or not used drugs.
2. *Factors contributing to use or abstinence.* The therapist asks the caregiver to describe factors that contributed to substance use or abstinence.
3. *New developments, questions or concerns, and homework.* The therapist describes to the caregiver information about the session that will help the caregiver support the ABC assessment process. The therapist might report, for example, newly discovered triggers or factors that helped the youth avoid drug use. The therapist asks for the caregiver's perspective on what was learned during the session and for questions or concerns. The therapist also describes the youth's new homework assignments and the caregiver's role in those assignments.

Permanent Caregiver Absence

With modifications, the ABC assessment component of CM treatment can be implemented in the context of individual treatment sessions with the youth alone. The therapist will be the youth's partner in all aspects of treatment. Thus, for each session checklist item and homework assignment, the therapist executes the behavior specified for the caregiver. To accurately identify and then change specific aspects of the youth's social and physical context that contribute to drug use, it might also be helpful to obtain the perspective of other individuals who are intimate with that context. The therapist does not live in the youth's everyday family, school, and peer contexts, and the youth is likely to detect only some of the factors in those contexts that are linked with drug use. In addition, the treatment might be more effective if someone other than the therapist can ensure the youth is positively reinforced after instances of nonuse and ensure that consequences follow instances of drug use. Therefore, if the youth's primary caregiver will not be available to participate in any part of the treatment process, the therapist is encouraged to obtain permission from the youth to contact other supportive adults (e.g., a relative, favorite teacher, coach) from the ecology and ask them to participate in treatment. If either agency policy or youth preference makes obtaining such permission difficult, the therapist can proceed without the benefit of external sources of information and support for the youth's treatment.

Self-Management Planning and Drug Refusal Skills Training (Chapter 5)

As noted previously, caregiver involvement in CM is usually critical for therapeutic success. Yet, despite the therapist's best efforts, such involvement is sometimes impossible to achieve consistently. In such cases, the following guidelines might be useful.

Temporary Caregiver Absence

When a caregiver is absent from the initial treatment session outlining the self-management or drug refusal planning processes, the therapist should be able to continue with the initial goals of the session, because most of the materials can be administered to the youth alone. However, the therapist conducting the initial self-management planning and drug refusal skills sessions with the youth alone has several additional responsibilities. These include:

1. *Before* starting the individual session with the youth, the therapist emphasizes the important role of the youth's caregiver in these plans.

2. *During* the sessions, the therapist refers to specific ways the caregiver can be involved in self-management and drug refusal skills development and asks the youth to give the caregiver feedback on these plans. The therapist might also ask the youth to role-play the process of giving such feedback to the caregiver.

3. *After* the session, the therapist should provide information to the caregiver about the self-management or drug refusal processes, ensure that the caregiver understands the plans, and cultivate caregiver engagement in the processes. The therapist should schedule a call with the caregiver as soon as possible to ensure that the caregiver understands and is willing to participate in the youth's self-management and drug refusal plans.

When the caregiver has attended the sessions that introduce the self-management and drug refusal planning processes but is unable to attend subsequent sessions, the therapist should contact the caregiver before and after the individual sessions with the youth. After the self-management planning sessions, the therapist should get the caregiver's perspective on the particular self-management tasks covered in the sessions. The therapist and caregiver can probably review and discuss each of the first four tasks associated with self-management by telephone with relatively little difficulty. The therapist should obtain the caregiver's perspective on (1) triggers that are particularly potent, (2) possible strategies for managing triggers that could be added to the list brainstormed by the therapist and youth, (3) a good strategy to be tried without exposing the youth to undue risk of use, and (4) rating the difficulty of the strategy the youth selected. The therapist should also describe the homework associated with the missed session and respond to any questions or concerns the caregiver has about the session and homework.

The latter tasks entailed in self-management planning (i.e., role-played practice and providing the youth with specific feedback on the role play), however, are more difficult to accomplish by telephone. When the caregiver has missed a session involving these tasks, the therapist can (1) describe the nature of the role play with the caregiver, (2) obtain the caregiver's perspective regarding how realistic the scenario seems to be, (3) and discuss possibilities for how best to practice the role plays and provide specific feedback at home before the next session. A similar process should be followed in contacting the caregiver after drug refusal skills training sessions.

Permanent Caregiver Absence

Permanent caregiver absence can impair the development and implementation of self-management and drug refusal plans. With only the youth's perspective available to accomplish self-management (e.g., trigger selection, brainstorming, strategy selection, and rating of strategy difficulty) and drug refusal planning, fewer strategies are likely to be generated, and some triggers for which management strategies are needed and ideas for refusal plans might be overlooked. Thus, when such planning occurs primarily in the context of individual treatment sessions with a youth, the therapist will need to take a more active role in the sessions. He or she should provide the kinds of ideas and guidance otherwise provided by a primary caregiver. For the final two tasks of the sessions (e.g., practice and feedback), therapists will need to rely more heavily on youth feedback concerning the feasibility of the strategies developed during the session. The therapist might work with the youth to identify individuals in his or her everyday life who can help the youth practice the self-management and drug refusal strategies and provide support for using them in real-life situations. Such individuals might include teachers, coaches, relatives, or neighbors. The therapist should set aside extra time to help the youth identify and access these social supports.

The Point-and-Level Reward System (Chapter 6)

If the therapist has not been able to successfully engage a primary caregiver in treatment during the ABC assessment (Chapter 4) and self-management planning and drug refusal skills training (Chapter 5) aspects of CM, efforts should be renewed to engage a caregiver in the Point-and-Level Reward System components of treatment. If these efforts fail, then the therapist should seek permission from the youth and caregiver to identify another adult who can be involved in the treatment process.

Temporary Caregiver Absence

When a caregiver who has previously attended treatment sessions misses the first session in which the point-and-level reward system is introduced, the following guidelines apply.

1. *Before* starting the explanation of the contract and point-and-level reward system, the therapist should emphasize the importance of the youth's caregiver in completing the contract and implementing the system.

2. *During* the session, the therapist should refer to specific ways the caregiver will be involved in the CM contract and point-and-level system. The therapist might describe the point system, introduce the contract, interview the youth about rewards and privileges he or she currently receives at home, and review the checkbook system with the youth alone. The therapist should not, however, finalize any aspects of the contract or *Reward Menu* (Form 6.3) until the caregiver is present. Given the complexity of the point system and the contractual nature of the contingency plan, caregiver presence in sessions with the therapist and youth will be required to complete these components of CM.

3. *After* the individual session with the youth, the therapist should quickly identify the barriers to caregiver attendance at the session and develop strategies to overcome them. In fact, the therapist might decide to end the session with the youth early to allow time to call the caregiver or speak to other adults who have accompanied the youth to the clinic. If the youth comes to the clinic twice in a row without a caregiver while developing the contract with point-and-level reward system component of CM, the therapist

should either halt CM and focus on engaging the caregiver in treatment or consider reviewing the ABC assessment and self-management plan sections until the caregiver can be reintegrated into the sessions.

After the caregiver understands the point-and-level system, has agreed to the rewards and consequences of drug use, and has signed the contract, his or her presence in treatment sessions is not absolutely essential *as long as the therapist and caregiver communicate* about the outcomes of drug testing and implementation of contingencies since the last session. Thus, the therapist can proceed with a youth alone to review progress with the point system as long as caregiver input is received for each session. Ideally, the therapist will communicate with the caregiver before the session with the youth, even if that means delaying the session while the therapist speaks with the caregiver on the telephone.

Permanent Caregiver Absence

When the youth's primary caregiver is not involved in treatment and another adult in the youth's natural ecology is not available to support the treatment process, CM strategies will need to be modified to resemble those proven to be effective with substance-abusing and substance-dependent adults. When treating youth in an individual therapy context, without the assistance of the family members, the therapist, rather than the caregiver, becomes the central person monitoring drug use and ensuring that drug screens are obtained and consequences are provided. Hence, the therapist, rather than the caregiver, takes on the role of observing, motivating, rewarding, and withholding rewards. Detailed suggestions and materials to assist the therapist in modifying the tasks of the point-and-level system and forms to better suit the needs of youth in treatment without family members are subsequently provided.

Drug Testing Protocol (Chapter 7)

Temporary Caregiver Absence

When a caregiver who has previously attended treatment sessions misses the first session in which the urine screens are introduced, the following guidelines apply.

1. *Before* starting the explanation of the urine drug testing process, the therapist emphasizes the importance of the youth's caregiver in this process.

2. *During* the session, the therapist refers to specific ways the caregiver will be involved in the urine testing process. The therapist might describe the process and how it will interface with the contingency contract. *The therapist should not, however, collect a specimen unless he or she has received assurance that the caregiver is ready to follow through with the consequences outlined in the contract based on the results of the test.*

3. *After* the individual session with the youth, the therapist should quickly contact the caregiver to identify the barriers to caregiver attendance at the session and develop strategies to overcome them. The therapist should communicate with the caregiver about the urine testing process and stress the importance of caregiver involvement in the overall

implementation of the program as well as in the sustainability of the interventions and outcomes. If the youth comes to the clinic twice in a row without a caregiver, the therapist should consider proceeding with on-site office drug testing *and follow up with the caregiver immediately to ensure that he or she follows through with the contingency contract.*

Permanent Caregiver Absence

When treating youth without caregiver involvement cannot be avoided, the therapist should collect all urine on site in the office bathroom. One special caveat is that the youth will only be able to be tested when he or she has an appointment. This will make collecting urine without the youth's prior knowledge impossible. As a result, the therapist should schedule appointments frequently enough to ensure drug detection. Strategies to accomplish rescheduling might include shifting sessions (e.g., Wednesday one week, Monday the next) or creating additional drop-in appointments for specimen collection. The youth should be informed that all missed urine collection appointments will be counted as dirty screens. Drugs with very short half-lives, such as alcohol, may not be amenable to CM treatment in the absence of a caregiver or supportive adult unless methods of testing are utilized that provide a window long enough to ensure most use is detected.

IMPLEMENTING THE CONTRACT WITH THE POINT-AND-LEVEL REWARD SYSTEM IN THE CONTEXT OF PERMANENT CAREGIVER ABSENCE

Although most CM components can be completed, albeit not optimally, by the therapist working individually with the adolescent, the contract with point-and-level reward system component presents special challenges, because it relies on privileges and rewards provided by the family. Consequently, additional guidance and materials are presented to facilitate the implementation of this important component of CM by therapists working individually with youth.

Materials

- *Point-and-Level System Contract for Individual Youth* (Form 9.1)
- *List of Potential Rewards for Individual Treatment* (Form 9.2)
- *List of Potential Rewards Example for Individual Treatment* (Handout 9.1)
- *Reward Menu Example for Individual Treatment* (Handout 9.2)

Therapist Task 1: Introducing the Point System to the Youth

A modified *Point-and-Level System Contract for Individual Youth* (Form 9.1) has been developed for use with an individual youth. Throughout the introduction of the point-and-level system (see *Therapist Checklist 6.1: Introducing the Point-and-Level System and Contract*), the therapist should modify the checklist such that the role of the therapist is substituted for the role of the caregiver. As described in the next section, the processes of identifying an MVP and of earning rewards other than money will be modified slightly, but will still take place. Prior to reading the contract with the youth, the therapist should discuss the importance of involving a supportive adult from the youth's natural ecology in the CM treatment to help provide social support, encouragement, and rewards when the youth has clean screens. The contract outlines the potential role this supportive adult might take in providing rewards. After reading and signing the contract, the therapist can help the youth identify adults in his or her ecology who might be involved in providing rewards. The therapist can consider asking these adults to provide reinforcers for the youth's abstinence if youth permission to contact such adults is given.

Use of Vouchers/Gift Certificates

When treating adolescents in an individual therapy context, without the assistance of family members, the therapist, rather than the caregiver, takes on the role of observing, motivating, rewarding, and withholding rewards. In this context, it is often helpful if the therapist has access to coupons, vouchers, or gift certificates to help reinforce abstinence. Methods of providing these resources have varied across studies with adults and youth (Higgins, Silverman, & Heil, 2007). Some methods of providing clinic-based rewards to facilitate CM treatment include:

- Providing assistance in purchasing items or services for clients such as shoes, clothing, a haircut, books, and sports equipment.
- Purchasing coupons or gift certificates to online stores, local stores, restaurants, movie theaters, bowling alleys, gas stations, and recreational facilities.
- Obtaining coupons or free tickets for fast food stores, toy stores, hair salons, parks, and other attractions.

When the therapist subsidizes abstinence, several key issues are important to monitor. First, the client should not receive cash directly as such might trigger substance use. Also, the therapist needs to follow up to ensure that the targeted item was actually obtained, perceived as rewarding, and not diverted to facilitate drug use. The therapist should clearly state the amount of money or coupons the client can earn (e.g., 100 dollars), and the *Reward Menu* (Form 6.3) should clearly specify the reimbursement rate (e.g., 1 point per dollar for music downloads) for vouchers.

Therapist Task 2: Developing Rewards for the Point-and-Level System

The central goals of this task remain the same as described in Chapter 6: to develop a list of rewards that can be used as incentives for the youth's abstinence. The key difference is that the rewards will need to be items that the therapist can provide or help make available to the youth. While items that can be purchased using vouchers, gift certificates, or donations provided by the clinic are obvious candidates for the list, the therapist has access to other valued resources that can be leveraged for treatment. These resources generally fall under the broad categories of "time" and "influence." With some creative thinking, the therapist and youth can develop a list of rewards (see *List of Potential Rewards Example for Individual Treatment* [Handout 9.1] for examples) using resources that will not cost the therapist money. Some examples of ways the therapist can wield influence (with signed consent from the youth) to reinforce abstinence include providing letters of recommendation, making calls to teachers or probation officers, making employment connections, and advocating for free goods or services for the youth. The therapist might also give time or other resources to reward abstinence. The therapist might be able to help with homework or job applications, provide access to a computer for word processing, be a source for borrowed books or for monitored access to the Internet, or spend more time with the youth in the session talking about something other than drug use. In addition, the therapist and youth should try to identify adults in the youth's ecology whom the youth is willing to involve in providing rewards. The therapist can consider asking these adults to provide reinforcers for the youth's abstinence if youth permission to contact such adults is provided. For example, a youth might consent for the therapist to speak with his uncle on the telephone (with youth present) for the purpose of engaging the uncle to provide a reward (e.g., taking the youth to dinner) when (and only when) the therapist calls and requests the reward. The final product of this work is written down on the *List of Potential Rewards for Individual Treatment* worksheet (Form 9.2), which serves as the groundwork for the reward menu.

The steps that follow are essentially the same as those used when working with caregivers (see *Therapist Checklist 6.2: Completing a Reward Menu*). That is, the therapist and youth identify an important privilege that can be administered following each clean drug screen and list it as the MVP. Then the therapist goes through the list and takes out any rewards that are counterproductive or inappropriate. At this point, the therapist works with the youth to assign points and considers placing some rewards under a different heading to reinforce another behavior (i.e., school attendance) if appropriate. When complete, the therapist has a working *Reward Menu* (Form 6.3). *Reward Menu Example for Individual Treatment* (Handout 9.2) provides an example of a menu that might be used in the absence of participating adults.

Therapist Task 3: Monitoring Points Earned and Exchanged in the Checkbook System

The primary difference in the implementation of this task and that described in Chapter 6 is that the youth completes all checkbook transactions in the office with the therapist. The therapist should keep a copy of the checkbook on file to avoid confusion if the youth forgets or attempts to alter records. Ideally, this task should occur at a regular time each week, after the validation of urine screen results.

Therapist Task 4: Reviewing and Revising the Point System in Subsequent Sessions

There are no substantial changes in this task. The therapist works directly with the youth to complete homework, provide feedback on assignments, address barriers to drug testing, assign rewards or consequences, and instill hope.

Therapist Task 5: Maintaining the Incentive System after Treatment Ends

This aspect of treatment is difficult to provide without the involvement of a caregiver or responsible adult in the youth's ecology. To increase the chances the system can be maintained after treatment, the therapist should search for someone in the youth's social network who can be engaged to assist with abstinence. Sometimes youth are more willing or able to find sources of interpersonal support when they have experienced success remaining drug free. Thus, caregivers, relatives, pastors, and friends the youth rejected as candidates for serving in the caregiver role at the beginning of treatment might now be viable options for helping him or her maintain abstinence after treatment ends. With the youth's written permission, this support person should be brought into the final planning sessions with the youth and therapist. Here the therapist can:

1. Review success.
2. Predict the youth's ability to sustain positive gains.
3. Put plans into place for dealing with relapse that utilize the support person.
4. Update the *Reward Menu* (Form 6.3) to identify privileges the youth will access either directly or through the support person when abstinent.
5. Develop a schedule for the youth to get urine screens.
6. Develop a plan for relapse, including what kinds of behaviors or events should signal the support person and youth that it is time to get additional help or return to therapy.

If an individual in the youth's natural ecology cannot be identified to ensure drug test collection, it is very unlikely that the youth will be tested and rewards provided for abstinence. Under such circumstances, the therapist can attempt to develop a contract with the youth to identify the signs that constitute relapse and the actions the youth will take when these signs appear. Often calling the therapist to re-enroll in treatment or to garner support may be an appropriate part of this plan.

THERAPIST FORMS AND HANDOUTS FOR CHAPTER 9: CONDUCTING CONTINGENCY MANAGEMENT WITHOUT CAREGIVERS

FORM 9.1

Point-and-Level System Contract for Individual Youth

We have agreed that helping you stop using drugs/alcohol is a very important job that needs to be done. This contract outlines what each of our roles will be in that work. It describes a plan by which you can earn points and privileges as a reward when you have clean urine screens and alcohol breath scans each week. You can trade in your points to your therapist or a supportive adult for rewards and privileges that we agree on. You will also earn a most valued privilege (MVP) from your therapist or a supportive adult each time that you have clean test results.

Now, here's more information about the point system (also see *Point-and-Level System at a Glance* [Handout 6.1]:

Level I (from start of treatment until 6 straight weeks of clean screens):

- You will receive 25 points *today* for starting the program. This will only happen once.
- Points can be traded for rewards.
- We will create a list of rewards you would like to earn, called a reward menu.
- Rewards can be activities (e.g., movies) or things you want (e.g., music).
- A urine drug screen will be conducted at least once a week, maybe more often. Alcohol breath scans will be conducted whenever your therapist thinks you might have been drinking.
- You will earn 12 points per week for clean urine drug screens and alcohol breath scans.
- If the drug screen and breath scan are negative (clean) you will be able to cash in some earned points for rewards.
- You will also get something called a most valued privilege, or MVP, from your therapist or supportive adult each time you have a clean urine screen and alcohol breath scan.
- We will work together to decide on an MVP that will help motivate you to stay clean.
- If the drug screen or breath scan is positive (dirty):
    - You will not earn points.
    - You will not earn your MVP until you test clean again.
    - You will not be able to purchase rewards until you test clean again.
- You will keep track of your points with a checkbook and write checks to your therapist or supportive adult to cash in points.
- You may only spend points when your most recent drug screen is clean.
- You may only spend points that you have already earned. In other words, you cannot go into debt in your checkbook or spend points you have not yet earned.

Level II (after 6 straight weeks of clean screens):

- When you have been clean for 6 weeks in a row, you will advance to Level II.
- In Level II, you will earn a total of 24 points (12 bonus points) for each week your screens are clean.
- Just like in Level I, you will earn your MVP and be able to write checks to spend points for rewards when your screens and scans are clean.
- If you have a dirty urine screen or breath scan while you are in Level II, you will drop back to Level I.
- You will have to test clean for 4 more weeks in a row to earn your way back to Level II again.

(cont.)

Level III (after 4 straight weeks of clean screens in Level II):

- Once you have tested clean for 4 straight weeks at Level II, you will advance to Level III.
- In Level III, you will work with your therapist and, if possible, a supportive adult, to figure out how to help you have continued success staying drug and alcohol free.
- You will develop a sobriety maintenance plan, which is a plan to help you stay clean in the future.

Your signature means that you agree to participate in this program.

Youth	Date	Supportive Adult	Date
Therapist	Date		

FORM 9.2

List of Potential Rewards for Individual Treatment

(For use only when caregiver absence from treatment is permanent)

Type of reward	What others might give

What I would like to purchase with vouchers (optional, if available)

What other adults might agree to provide

(cont.)

Type of reward	What others might give
Therapist time resources	
Therapist influence resources	

HANDOUT 9.1

List of Potential Rewards Example for Individual Treatment

(For use only when caregiver absence from treatment is permanent)

Type of reward	What others might give
What I would like to purchase with vouchers (optional, if available)	
Clothing	Therapist—vouchers
Music player	Therapist—vouchers
What other adults might agree to provide	
Weight-lifting supplies	Older brother might give his old set to me
Go to work with uncle	Uncle Joe might let me work in his repair shop
Lunch	Uncle Joe might buy me lunch

(cont.)

List of Potential Rewards Example for Individual Treatment *(page 2 of 2)*

Type of reward	What others might give
Therapist time resources	
Job	Help me fill out applications
	Let me use computer to complete applications
	Let me use Internet to look up jobs
	Help me find a good job
School	Help me with my homework
	Let me use computer to do my reports
	Help me find books/references for reports
Other	Ask my probation officer to leave me alone
	Help me look up weight-lifting info on Internet
Therapist influence resources	
Job	Ask someone to hire me
School	Tell my guidance counselor how good I am doing
Other	Tell my stepfather I am working the program

HANDOUT 9.2

Reward Menu Example for Individual Treatment

(For use only when caregiver absence from treatment is permanent)

Type of reward	What others might give
MVP: Free food—option A	Therapist will supply free fast food coupon with each clean screen.
-or-	Therapist—vouchers
MVP: Lunch with uncle—option B	Uncle will provide lunch on the weekend after therapist calls to report clean screen.

Vouchers

Clothing	1 point = $1 in vouchers
Music player/tunes	1 point = $1 in vouchers

What other adults might provide with call from therapist

Weight-lifting supplies	7 points = set of two weights (i.e., two 10-lb plates) 10 points = gloves and belt 20 points = weight bar 50 points = weight bench Brother has been called with consent and agrees to provide these items after therapist calls to prompt him.
Go to work with uncle	7 points = work with Uncle Joe in car repair shop one weekend day from 9 A.M. to 12 P.M. after therapist calls to prompt him.

(cont.)

Type of reward	What others might give
Therapist time resources	
Job	5 points = 30 minutes of help with job applications
	5 points = 30 minutes of computer or Internet time for job search
	5 points = 30 minutes of help making a job plan
School	5 points = 30 minutes of help with homework
	5 points = 30 minutes of computer time for homework
	5 points = 30 minutes of help finding books/references
Other	10 points = 30 minutes of Internet time for approved weight-lifting sites
Therapist influence resources	
Job	10 weeks straight clean, therapist to write letter of reference for youth (w/consent)
School	8 weeks straight clean, therapist to write letter to school for the youth (w/consent)
Other	12 weeks straight clean, therapist to write letter to probation officer and call (w/consent)
	4 weeks straight clean, therapist to call stepfather with youth consent and youth present to discuss youth's progress in treatment

References

American Association for Clinical Chemistry. (1988). Critical issues in urinalysis of abused substances: Report of the Substance Abuse Testing Committee. *Clinical Chemistry, 34*, 605–632.

Azrin, N. H., Acierno, R., Kogan, E., Donohue, B., Besalel, V., & McMahon, P. T. (1996). Follow-up results of supportive versus behavioral therapy for illicit drug abuse. *Behaviour Research and Therapy, 34*, 41–46.

Azrin, N. H., Donohue, B., Besalel, V. A., Kogan, E. S., & Acierno, R. (1994). Youth drug abuse treatment: A controlled outcome study. *Journal of Child and Adolescent Substance Abuse, 3*, 1–16.

Azrin, N. H., McMahon, P. T., Donohue, B., Besalel, V., Lapinski, K. J., Kogan, E., et al. (1994). Behavioral therapy for drug abuse: A controlled treatment outcome study. *Behavioral Research and Therapy, 32*, 857–866.

Bickel, W. K., Amass, L., Higgins, S. T., Badger, G. J., & Esch, R. A. (1997). Effects of adding behavioral treatment to opioid detoxification with buprenorphine. *Journal of Consulting and Clinical Psychology, 65*, 803–810.

Brown, S. A., Myers, M. G., Mott, M. A., & Vik, P. W. (1994). Correlates of success following treatment for adolescent substance abuse. *Applied and Preventive Psychology, 3*, 61–73.

Budney, A. J., & Higgins, S. T. (1998). *A community reinforcement plus vouchers approach: Treating cocaine addiction* (NIH Publication No. 98-4309). Rockville, MD: National Institute on Drug Abuse.

Center for Substance Abuse Treatment. (1999). *Treatment of substance use disorders among adolescents* (Treatment Improvement Protocol Series 3, K. C. Winters, Ed.). Rockville, MD: Author.

Cunningham, P. B., Donohue, B., Randall, J., Swenson, C. C., Rowland, M. D., Henggeler, S. W., et al. (2002). *Integrating contingency management into multisystemic therapy*. Charleston: Family Services Research Center, Medical University of South Carolina.

Cunningham, P. B., Schoenwald, S. K., Rowland, M. D., Swenson, C. C., Henggeler, S. W., Randall, J., et al. (2004). *Implementing contingency management for adolescent substance abuse in outpatient settings*. Charleston: Family Services Research Center, Department of Psychiatry and Behavioral Sciences, Medical University of South Carolina.

Davis, M., Eshelman, E. R., & McKay, M. (2000). *The relaxation & stress reduction workbook*. Oakland, CA: New Harbinger.

Dodge, K. A., Dishion, T. J., & Lansford, J. E. (Eds.). (2006). *Deviant peer influences in programs for youth: Problems and solutions*. New York: Guilford Press.

Donohue, B., & Azrin, N. H. (2001). Family behavior therapy. In E. F. Wagner & H. B. Waldron

(Eds.), *Innovations in adolescent substance abuse interventions* (pp. 205–227). New York: Pergamon Press.

D'Zurilla, T. J., & Nezu, A. M. (1999). *Problem-solving therapy: A social competence approach to clinical intervention* (2nd ed.). New York: Springer.

Eddy, J. M., & Chamberlain, P. (2000). Family management and deviant peer association as mediators of the impact of treatment condition on youth antisocial behavior. *Journal of Consulting and Clinical Psychology, 68*, 857–863.

Family Services Research Center. (2008a). *Implementing contingency management for adolescent substance abuse in outpatient settings* (2nd ed.). Charleston: Family Services Research Center, Department of Psychiatry and Behavioral Sciences, Medical University of South Carolina.

Family Services Research Center. (2008b). *Implementing contingency management for adolescent substance abuse in outpatient settings: Drug court version.* Charleston: Family Services Research Center, Department of Psychiatry and Behavioral Sciences, Medical University of South Carolina.

Henggeler, S. W., Chapman, J. E., Rowland, M. D., Halliday-Boykins, C. A., Randall, J., Shackelford, J., et al. (2007). If you build it, they will come: Statewide practitioner interest in CM for youths. *Journal of Substance Abuse Treatment, 32*, 121–131.

Henggeler, S. W., Chapman, J. E., Rowland, M. D., Halliday-Boykins, C. A., Randall, J., Shackelford, J., et al. (2008). Statewide adoption and initial implementation of contingency management for substance abusing adolescents. *Journal of Consulting and Clinical Psychology, 76*, 556–567.

Henggeler, S. W., Halliday-Boykins, C. A., Cunningham, P. B., Randall, J., Shapiro, S. B., & Chapman, J. E. (2006). Juvenile drug court: Enhancing outcomes by integrating evidence-based treatments. *Journal of Consulting and Clinical Psychology, 74*(1), 42–54.

Henggeler, S. W., McCart, M. R., Cunningham, P. B., & Chapman, J. E. (2011). *Enhancing the effectiveness of juvenile drug courts by integrating evidence-based practices.* Manuscript submitted for publication.

Henggeler, S. W., Pickrel, S. G., Brondino, M. J., & Crouch, J. L. (1996). Eliminating (almost) treatment dropout of substance abusing or dependent delinquents through home-based multisystemic therapy. *American Journal of Psychiatry, 153*, 427–428.

Henggeler, S. W., & Sheidow, A. J. (2011). Empirically supported family-based treatments for conduct disorder and delinquency. *Journal of Marital and Family Therapy.*

Henggeler, S. W., Sheidow, A. J., Cunningham, P. B., Donohue, B. C., & Ford, J. D. (2008). Promoting the implementation of an evidence-based intervention for adolescent marijuana abuse in community settings: Testing the use of intensive quality assurance. *Journal of Clinical Child and Adolescent Psychology, 37*, 682–689.

Higgins, S. T., & Budney, A. J. (1993). Treatment of cocaine dependence through the principles of behavior analysis and behavioral pharmacology. In L. S. Onken, J. D. Blaine, & J. J. Boren (Eds.), *Behavioral treatments for drug abuse and dependence* (National Institute on Drug Abuse Research Monograph 137, NIH Pub. No. 93-3684, pp. 97–121). Rockville, MD: National Institute on Drug Abuse.

Higgins, S. T., Sigmon, S. C., Wong, C. J., Heil, S. H., Badger, G. J., Donham, R., et al. (2003). Community reinforcement therapy for cocaine dependent outpatients. *Archives of General Psychiatry, 60*, 1043–1052.

Higgins, S. T., Silverman, K., & Heil, S. H. (2007). *Contingency management in substance abuse treatment.* New York: Guilford Press.

Huey, S. J., Henggeler, S. W., Brondino, M. J., & Pickrel, S. G. (2000). Mechanisms of change in multisystemic therapy: Reducing delinquent behavior through therapist adherence and improved family and peer functioning. *Journal of Consulting and Clinical Psychology, 68*, 451–467.

Johnston, L. D., O'Malley, P. M., Bachman, J. G., & Schulenberg, J. E. (2007). *Monitoring the Future national survey results on drug use, 1975–2006: Vol. I. Secondary school students* (NIH Pub. No. 07-6205). Bethesda, MD: National Institute on Drug Abuse.

Liberman, A. M. (Ed.). (2008). *The long view of crime: A synthesis of longitudinal research*. New York: Springer.

Loeber, R., Farrington, D. P., Stouthamer-Loeber, M., & Van Kammen, W. B. (1998). *Antisocial behavior and mental health problems: Explanatory factors in childhood and adolescence*. Mahwah, NJ: Erlbaum.

Mayfield, D., McLead, G., & Hall, P. (1974). The CAGE Questionnaire. *American Journal of Psychiatry, 131*, 1121–1128.

Munger, R. (1998). *The ecology of troubled children: Changing children's behavior by changing the places, activities, and people in their lives*. Brookline, MA: Brookline Books.

National Institute on Drug Abuse. (2009). *Principles of drug addiction treatment: A research-based guide* (2nd ed.) (NIH Pub. No. 09-4180). Rockville, MD: U.S. Department of Health and Human Services, National Institutes of Health.

Petry, N. M. (2000). A comprehensive guide to the application of contingency management procedures in clinical settings. *Drug and Alcohol Dependence, 58*, 9–25.

Petry, N. M., Martin, B., Cooney, J. L., & Kranzler, H. R. (2000). Give them prizes and they will come: Contingency management for treatment of alcohol dependence. *Journal of Consulting and Clinical Psychology, 68*, 250–257.

Roozen, H. G., Boulogne, J. J., van Tulder, M. W., van den Brink, W., De Jong, C. A., & Kerkhof, A. J. (2004). A systematic review of the effectiveness of the community reinforcement approach in alcohol, cocaine and opioid addiction. *Drug and Alcohol Dependence, 74*(1), 1–13.

Schaeffer, C. M., Chang, R., & Henggeler, S. W. (2009). Responding to use of illicit drugs. In K. Geldard (Ed.), *Practical interventions for young people at risk* (pp. 134–144). Thousand Oaks, CA: Sage.

Schaeffer, C. M., Henggeler, S. W., Chapman, J. E., Halliday-Boykins, C. A., Cunningham, P. B., Randall, J., et al. (2010). Mechanisms of effectiveness in juvenile drug court: Altering risk processes associated with delinquency and substance abuse. *Drug Court Review, 7*, 57–94.

Stanger, C., & Budney, A. J. (2010). Contingency management approaches for adolescent substance use disorders. *Child and Adolescent Psychiatric Clinics of North America, 19*, 547–562.

Stanger, C., Budney, A. J., Kamon, J. L., & Thostensen, J. (2009). A randomized trial of contingency management for adolescent marijuana abuse and dependence. *Drug and Alcohol Dependence, 105*, 240–247.

Tarter, R. E., Vanyukov, M., & Kirisci, L. (2008). Etiology of substance use disorder: Developmental perspective. In Y. Kaminer & O. G. Bukstein (Eds.), *Adolescent substance abuse: Psychiatric comorbidity and high-risk behaviors* (pp. 5–27). New York: Routledge.

Thomas, D. W. (1990). *Substance abuse screening protocol for the juvenile courts*. Pittsburgh: National Center for Juvenile Justice.

Waldron, H. B., & Turner, C. W. (2008). Evidence-based psychosocial treatments for adolescent substance abuse. *Journal of Clinical Child and Adolescent Psychology, 37*(1), 238–261.

Weisz, J. R., & Kazdin, A. E. (Eds.). (2010). *Evidence-based psychotherapies for children and adolescents* (2nd ed.). New York: Guilford Press.

Williams, R. J., & Chang, S. Y. (2000). A comprehensive and comparative review of adolescent substance abuse treatment outcome. *Clinical Psychology: Science and Practice, 7*(2), 138–166.

Winters, K. C., Latimer, W. W., & Stinchfield, R. (2001). Assessing adolescent substance use. In E. F. Wagner & H. B. Waldron (Eds.), *Innovations in adolescent substance abuse interventions* (pp. 1–29). New York: Pergamon.

Index

Page numbers followed by a *t* indicate tables.

H

I

L

M

N

O

P

R